Community Psychiatric Nursing

CARING FOR THE MI
HANDICAPPED IN TI

Patrick J. Carr
B.A. (Hons.), Ph.D., R.M.N., S.R.N.
Principal Lecturer; Head of Nursing Studies, Manchester Polytechinc

C. A. Butterworth
M.Sc., S.R.N., R.M.N., D.N.(London), Teacher's Certificate, Manchester University,
R.N.T.
Principal Lecturer in Nursing Studies, Manchester Polytechnic

B. E. Hodges
B.A.(Hons.), S.R.N., R.N.M.S., D.N.,(London), Teachers' Certificate,
Manchester University, R.N.T.
Senior Lecturer in Nursing Studies, Manchester Polytechnic

Foreword by
S. Moore
S.R.N., R.M.N., R.N.T.
Principal Nursing Officer, Department of Health and Social Security, London

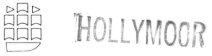

CHURCHILL LIVINGSTONE
EDINBURGH LONDON AND NEW YORK 1980

CHURCHILL LIVINGSTONE
Medical Division of Longman Group Limited

Distributed in the United States of America by
Churchill Livingstone Inc., 19 West 44th Street, New York,
N.Y. 10036 and by associated companies, branches and
representatives throughout the world.

First published 1980
  Reprinted 1982

ISBN 0 443 01550 3

British Library Cataloguing in Publication Data

Carr, P. J.
  Community psychiatric nursing.
  1. Psychiatric nursing—Great Britain—History
  2. Community mental health services—Great
  Britain—History
  3. Community health nursing—Great Britain—
  History
  I. Title   II. Butterworth, C. A.   III. Hodges, B. E.
  362.2'0425   RC440   79-40193

Printed in Singapore by Huntsmen Offset Printing Pte Ltd.

This book is dedicated with love to our wives—
Jennifer, Jacqueline and Mary—without whose indulgence
the work would never have been completed.

Foreword

The contribution which the community psychiatric nursing service is making to the total requirement in a comprehensive psychiatric service is considerable. Although the service was pioneered some 25 years ago, it is only in recent years that a significant expansion has taken place.

This is to some extent due to the reorganisation of the National Health Service and the consequent development along the lines of district service provision. On this basis a reduction of in-patient places is compensated for in the provision of alternative modes of service, e.g. day hospital, a wider range of social services residential care, as well as a community psychiatric nursing service. The change of emphasis to a district service provision has identified not only the essential need but the way in which community psychiatric nursing fits naturally into the pattern. It is involved with all the other elements of a comprehensive psychiatric service as indeed they are with it. The community psychiatric nursing service may act as the means to which social services and primary care medical and nursing services, the voluntary agencies and their services may be woven together as a complete therapeutic fabric serving the requirements of the individual at each particular phase in their illness.

Although community psychiatric nursing has made, and will continue to make, an invaluable contribution to what might be called the traditional service, it is in the developing District Psychiatric Service where the real potential has become apparent. No District Psychiatric Service is complete without this essential element. In fact there is an increasing concern by authorities to invest in a community psychiatric nursing service as an early priority in district development.

It is all the more important, therefore, that for an aspect of service which has a wide range of application, spanning the traditional existing service and the developing district service providing specialised service in its own professional right, there should be a work of reference available to the ever increasing number of professionals either directly or indirectly involved.

This book traces the conception, birth and development of this aspect of the psychiatric nursing service, pointing consistently to serving the particular needs of the patient whilst conveying the tremendous personal and professional satisfaction to be achieved by those delivering such a service. It identifies the increasing quality of service to be achieved by the provision of appropriate consideration for the individual patient in the particular place at the appropriate time, highlighting the vital importance of the most efficient use of a service resource such as specialised nursing manpower.

Because the word 'community' prefixes psychiatric nursing, there is a tendency to forget that the community psychiatric nursing service bridges the whole range of available psychiatric service whether at in-patient, day patient, out-patient or in provision of domiciliary support to the patient and/or the family. It contributes to the whole range of the district psychiatric services and makes available specialist professional advice to consultant psychiatrists, general practitioners, health visitors, district nurses, social workers and voluntary agencies.

This work is an important 'first' and although the authors modestly state it is 'but a starting point in the debate on community psychiatric nursing' it provides the range of necessary material upon which to understand the beginnings, to see the potentiality of contribution and to look to the horizon of increasing future possibility.

The publication of this book is a fitting tribute to the pioneers both the dreamers and the doers in the field of professional nursing education and the efficient delivery of service to those who need it. At the same time it retains a very practical flavour of common sense approach which in the present state of development of this service is fundamental to the preservation of flexibility in application.

The presentation of care studies is particularly helpful in understanding the principle which the text attempts to convey and the indications which are identified and point to the developing/ extending role of the psychiatric nurse, highlights many aspects of what is already an ongoing debate within the psychiatric nursing profession.

It is gratifying to see mental illness and mental handicap nursing dealt with in one volume but at the same time making appropriate distinction and similarity in the role of community psychiatric nursing in each service.

The range of references provided at the end of each chapter is considerable and these in themselves provide much useful follow-up material which the enthusiastic professionals will no doubt use to widen their background. This book will provide for an ever increasing need and many will find it deals effectively with an aspect of psychiatric nursing which in its present developmental state, is opportune.

1979   S.M.

Acknowledgements

We wish to record our thanks to the following organisations who have permitted us to use illustrations or quotations from their publications:

Constable and Co., Ltd., London.
Department of Health and Social Security Publications, London.
William Heinemann Medical Books Ltd., London.
Macmillan Publishing Co., Inc., New York.
Methuen and Co., Ltd., London.
Oxford University Press, Oxford.
Viking Penguin, Inc., New York.
John Wiley and Sons, New York.

Preface

This book was written in response to the need for a text in the field of community psychiatric nursing. The care of the mentally ill/handicapped in the community by nurses is a field of endeavour which is remarkable both for the speed at which it has developed, and the manner in which it has brought true practitioner status to nurses working in this challenging, new area. Services continue to make rapid progress—progress such that it is now possible to believe that in the near future many community psychiatric nursing services will have more patients on their books than their large, traditional, parent hospital. The role of the C.P.N.—already researched, and underpinned by post-basic training courses—is constantly being expanded by the diversity of service conditions encountered; this wide experience is, in turn, being consolidated through the medium of the C.P.N.A.—the professional association that exists for C.P.N.s.

That such a movement should have occurred is due to many factors, not least amongst which is the wave of humanism, generated in the main by behavioural scientists, which has swept through mental health/handicap in recent years. This has tended to bring to the fore a person sadly neglected by traditional, institutional psychiatry/mental handicap, viz. the patient. Serving the needs of the patient rather than those of the practitioner—of whatever calling, must be the prime focus of the N.H.S. Community psychiatric nursing is dedicated to this goal—in fact, the ultimate objective of the C.P.N. is to cater for the needs of the patient/client/person when they arise and in such a way as to prevent illness behaviour.

This book should therefore be of interest, not only to C.P.N.s, but to all those who participate in the care of the mentally ill/handicapped in the community—doctors (including G.P.s), nurses, psychologists and social workers.

It may also interest the nursing profession in general to see the way that C.P.N.s are using their expanded practitioner role. The legal outline, discussed in Chapter 8, is generally of use to all nurses. Patients and their relatives, and Community Health Councils may be interested to discover the range and scope that community psychiatric nursing has already achieved.

This book is but a starting-point in the debate on community psychiatric nursing: we seek not to define but to describe! If the reader is displeased by any inaccuracies, misinterpretation, mistakes or omissions which may have crept into the text we crave not your indulgence but your help in setting the record straight.

Manchester, August 1978   P.C.

Contents

1

Historical introduction

MENTAL NURSING

Histories of mental illness/psychiatry/institutions are almost always totally devoid of any reference to mental nursing. It is as if we never existed such is the silence on the subject.

Walk(1) begins his history with St. Vincent de Paul and Ste. Louise de Marillac in seventeenth century Paris. The institutions in which their respective orders worked—St. Lazare and the Petites-Maisons—became places where both the mentally ill, and those whom we would today describe as psychopathic personalities, were cared for on a 'moral model' basis (cf. Chapter 7). The seventeenth century is a good enough place to start, for it marked the end of the attitude of the middle ages to mental illness—typified by Galenic medicine, magic and sin, herb women, the obscurer healing arts, spirit-manipulation and illness, and witchcraft (cf. Clarke(2))—and it also signalled the beginning of a new era in psychiatry, one which was to be characterised by change and reconstruction. (The reconstruction was to culminate in the building of the large county asylums in the nineteenth century which, as Skultans(3) has noted, permitted 'the insane, particularly the pauper insane to be gradually separated from the destitute and the criminal'.)

The beginning of the new era was marked in a material way as follows: 'One of the social-psychiatric trends starting in the seventeenth century was the growth of privately owned madhouses' (Clarke 2). In keeping with the 'moral' climate which was strongly to pervade psychiatry for several hundred years and against which we are still fighting today, was the notion that mad people should be confined—as Foucault(4) has noted, definitions of madness always reflect a society's current notions on sanity etc. These private madhouses became somewhat notorious, as Jones(5) has remarked: 'In 1763, the general public was alarmed by revelations concerning the conditions in private madhouses and a movement to obtain statutory control was initiated'.

This, together with two other factors was to initiate the reform movement, as indicated by Jones. She names the other two factors as:

1. The Vagrancy Act, 1744; and
2. The fact that the King (George III) was known to be suffering from mental illness, which continued until he died in 1820.

The alarm generated by conditions in the private madhouses found expression in the Act for Regulating Private Madhouses, 1774.

It was in this sort of climate that mental nursing as we know it came into being. St. Vincent de Paul and Ste. Louise de Marillac have been mentioned already; their compatriots Philippe Pinel and Jean-Baptiste Pussin (the archetypal divisional nursing officer—psychiatry), also deserve special mention for their oft-quoted and well-known moral treatment of each patient, which allowed the chains of the Bicêtre and the Salpétrière to be cast aside in favour of more humane regimes. Walk(1) notes that: 'In England at this time there was no tradition of nursing either by religious communities or by recruits drawn from among former patients' (Pussin had himself been a patient at the Bicêtre, and it became his policy to recruit 'gardiens' from recovered or convalescent patients).

Jones(5) however, remarks that:

> The improvement in the public attitude to insanity was paralleled in three cities—London, Manchester and York—by the setting up of institutions where treatment of a relatively humane nature could be provided. St. Luke's Hospital, London was founded in 1751, the Manchester Lunatic Hospital in 1763 and the York Retreat in 1792. In these three cities was laid the foundation of the nineteenth century lunacy legislation.

Before lunacy reform took place on a national scale, there were some figures of note in mental nursing, mostly associated with the above three hospitals—Katherine Allen and her husband George Jepson, who became the first matron and chief male nurse of the Retreat when opened in 1796; Thomas Digby an attendant at St. Luke's Hospital who took charge of the first specially built asylum in Australia; and Mrs Ellis of the Wakefield and Middlesex asylums respectively. These people must be regarded as among the fathers and mothers of mental nursing in this country. They would not, of course, have been regarded as 'nurses'— they were much more likely referred to as 'keeper', 'attendant' or 'superintendent', the word 'nurse' where used at all, being reserved for women. The terms 'attendant' and 'superintendent' have of course survived to the present day—the author has often been addressed by patients as 'attendant' and the word 'superintendent' was still widely used in the N.H.S. until quite recently. (Salmon and N.H.S. re-organisation lessened it quite considerably.)

The County Asylum Act, 1808 (which became known as 'Wynn's

Act'), gave powers to local magistrates to build county asylums out of local rates. In twenty years, only nine counties proceeded to erect such asylums (cf. Jones(5)). It was a caring act, in that it sought to remove mentally ill people from gaols, houses of correction, poor houses and houses of industry, and confine them in a proper place—but it did begin the great containment of the mentally ill. There were enlightened people about to care for them—we have mentioned the nurses above; on the medical front, the Tukes, especially Samuel, at the Retreat and John Conolly at the Middlesex Asylum at Hanwell, did much to engender properly therapeutic attitudes towards patients—but after all is said and done, people were still being locked up, often on the most flimsy of grounds. The Lunatics Act of 1845, set the seal on the initial period of reform: 'The 1845 Act marked the culmination of a slow process of social evolution which transformed the "lunatics or mad persons" of 1744, into the "persons of unsound mind" of 1845' (Jones(5)). The Act completed the Lunacy Law structure—Lunacy Commissioners were named, and institutions of all types came under their inspection and supervision.

Thus the era of the attendant—as opposed to the keeper—had arrived. Yet his lot could not have been a very happy one. A tremendous expansion of the asylum service took place in the nineteenth century, but in the process the attendants' conditions of work, remuneration and status were left sadly behind, and training was virtually non-existent. It is undoubtedly true that Conolly tried to train his staff at Hanwell, particularly in the use of the 'no-restraint' system; that the first-known formal course of lectures given to mental nurses were delivered by Sir Alexander Morison at the Surrey Asylum; that W. A. F. Browne had in 1854 given a course of thirty lectures whose content was quite visionary to officers and attendants at Crichton Royal—but all this was very piecemeal. (It was quite amazing, as Walk(1) points out, that Florence Nightingale took no interest in the training of mental nurses.)

It was not until 1890, as Goddard(6) has noted, that any uniform training for mental nurses came into existence. It did so via the Royal Medico-Psychological Association (founded in 1841 as the Medico-Psychological Association). The first examination was held in May 1891, and certificates were granted to the successful candidates (all Scots). The course was of two years' duration, and included study of anatomy and physiology, psychology, mental diseases and the nursing of the insane, and some general nursing. There were lectures, clinical instruction and practical exercises. By the turn of the century, five to six hundred certificates were being granted every year. In 1908, the R.M.P.A. revised the curriculum to three years, with an intermediate exam at the end of the first year. The curriculum was thus brought into line with that which was in use in the general hospitals—an absurd anachronism which has persisted right down until the present day, and which led to an even worse disaster viz. 'the hospitalisation of the asylums'.

At the end of this time, two other events occurred which had implications for the development of mental nursing:

1. The Lunacy Act of 1890 became law, requiring an order from a Justice of the Peace for certification. Greene(7) remarks as follows:

> Unfortunately Parliament was busy undoing all the attempts to get national professional recognition of mental nurses by passing a series of laws such as the 1890 Lunacy Act, which had the effect of bringing the asylums under the control of the county councils.

In fact, the 1890 Act continued the county system of control which was quite inimical to the development of a national unitary professional group.

2. In 1896, the Asylum Workers Association was born, and worked vigorously to improve the lot of attendants. After twenty years of lobbying, in 1909 the Asylum Officers' Superannuation Act was at last passed. Unfortunately the Act was not quite what had been wanted, causing members to resign from the A.W.A. and found a trades union—the National Asylum Workers Union (N.A.W.U.) (The Mental Hospital and Institutional Workers Union(8)). Their aims were more service-orientated than those of the A.W.A., less concerned with status and training, more concerned with improving conditions and hours of work, and regulating conditions between employers. There has got to be a moral in there somewhere!

After a great deal of inter-necine strife on the question of State Registration of nurses, and, so far as mental nurses were concerned involving the Medico-Psychological Association (M.P.A.), the Royal British Nurses Association (R.B.N.A.)—formed by Mrs Bedford Fenwick in 1889, and greatly prejudiced against asylum-trained nurses—and the Asylum Workers Association (A.W.A.), it came to pass that the Nurses' Registration Act of 1919 contained provision for 'nurses trained in the nursing and care of persons suffering from mental diseases'. The N.A.W.U. nominated Mr T. Christian and Nurse N. Wooster to serve on the G.N.C. Council, and Mr Christian from Banstead was duly elected and was present when the G.N.C. for England and Wales met for the first time in May, 1920. The fighting had not finished, however, as Walk(1) reminds us:

> In the same year (1923), a joint conference was held between the Council, the Association and the Board of Control. It was there stated on behalf of the Council that it was realised that mental nurses would for a

considerable time to come, prefer not to register and therefore the examination and certificate of the Association would be necessary as before. The Council welcomed the assistance of the M.P.A. and invited the Association to nominate examiners and to appoint an advisory committee to the Council.

This situation existed until 1951 when mental nursing was finally fully integrated with other types of nursing under a reorganized statutory body.

Whilst all this fighting was going on—the actual training of course changed little, if at all—there were significant statutory developments in the field of mental health:

1. The Mental Treatment Act, 1930, which introduced two new categories of patient who might be received without certification, *viz.* 'voluntary' patients, who might leave after giving seventy-two hours notice, having entered hospital of their own volition of course, and 'temporary' patients, who might be expected to gain the power of volition within six months. The Act recognised the changes that had occurred in the field, and therefore re-organised the Board of Control, provided for out-patient clinics, brought terminology into the twentieth century, and generally gave fresh impetus to the mental health movement.

2. The National Health Service Act 1946, which of course, set up the health service. The term 'certified', 'voluntary' and 'temporary' were retained, but the treatment of the mentally ill and handicapped was seen in the same context as the treatment of the physically ill and handicapped. All hospitals apart from a few such as the Retreat and Cheadle Royal (the former Manchester Lunatic Hospital)—in fact two of the three hospitals which led the way to nineteenth century lunacy legislation—now became responsible to the Minister of Health.

3. The Mental Health Act 1959, sought to give expression to the tremendous potential for change which had come about in the 'fifties', due mainly to the work of bio-chemists and behavioural scientists. Old terminology disappeared to be replaced by new. A platform was created for the development of community care. But resources—both human in the shape of social workers and local health and welfare personnel, and material in the sense of community accommodation and training of personnel—were sadly lacking; the therapeutic potential especially of the nurses was never realised.

The Act is now sorely lacking in many areas, not least of which are the rights, status and place of mental and mental handicap nurses in the therapeutic team.

4. The N.H.S. Re-organisation Act, 1974, completed the 'hospitalisation of mental nursing'!

In the last hundred years then, the lot of the mental nurse has varied.

So far as conditions of service are concerned, there have clearly been substantial improvements and union activity has obviously played a large part in this; so far as training, education and professional status are concerned the improvements have been minimal, due to the historical lack of interest in these areas shown by the unions, and the ineffectiveness/disinterest of professional bodies such as the A.W.A. and R.C.N. (It is after all within living memory that the R.C.N. admitted mental nurses to membership!)

Overall the mental nurse has gone through quite a range of titles and functions:

1. When all seemed darkness in the middle ages, it was the nuns who cared for both the physically and mentally ill
—the Order of the Holy Ghost founded in 1145 staffed many medieval hospitals and probably even undertook training activities; the Hospital Sisters of the Mercy of Jesus, founded around the same time, also looked after the insane.

2. The monks followed up this tradition
—the first asylum for the insane was founded in Valencia in 1409 by a Spanish monk, Juan Gilbert Joffre; The Brothers of Charity, notably at Charenton, cared for the insane; The Order of St. Vincent de Paul, as mentioned, was also very active in the field of mental health.

3. The next phase was that of keeper, who often treated the insane with great cruelty, and was far removed from the traditions of humanity begun by the nuns and monks.

4. Following on the heels of the keeper, came the attendant, who was to act as a kind of prison warder in the private madhouses and the asylums, both county and other.

5. With nursing registration, we became nurses, although our function changed little.

So, finally—what next? What is the next phase (title and function), for the mental nurse? We hope that as the pages of this book unfold before your eyes, you will gain an impression of where we are going next! In the final chapter, we shall make so bold as to suggest a direction—you may or may not agree! We shall see!

All that has been said is applicable equally to both mental and mental handicap nurses, perhaps more so to the latter, because no differentiation was made between the insane and the idiot/imbecile until this century in terms of care, and therefore no differentiation between those who did the caring. Legislation this century did begin a process of separation, and a discussion of this and its antecedents now follows.

Mental handicap nursing

Historically, the most severely handicapped were recognised first, and those that survived infancy would be cared for at home. Those people unable to support themselves would be accommodated in the only institutions, the workhouses and infirmaries provided under the Elizabethan poor law. Here, the intention was to provide a life-style inferior than the poorest farm labourers in order to discourage admission.

A phase of optimism was entered upon following the work of Itard (1801) and Sequin with their efforts at education of mentally handicapped people, culminating in the founding of the Park House at Highgate which proudly announced 'The Idiot may be educated', and the training colonies at Darenth Park, Starcross and Lancaster.

The phase changed to one of pessimism with the fears of 'national degeneracy' expressed by Mary Dendy and the Eugenics Society around the turn of the century when several occurrences coincided— the work of Binet on intelligence testing, Galton and the study of genetics, and the family studies of Goddard and Dugdale seeming to show that the mentally handicapped had more children and would thereby dilute the race. Segregation seemed the sensible policy. Mary Dendy of Cheshire stated that only permanent care would be efficacious in stemming the tide of feebleness of the mind, and at Stoke Park Colony Bristol it was stated that the care to be provided would be permanent and no-one would be knowingly admitted on a temporary basis. (They were of course right—some of them are still there.)

The segregation policy was endorsed by the 1913 Mental Deficiency Act.

In 1924 a committee was set up in order to ascertain:
1. How many defectives.
2. Best way of training them.

The report in 1929(9) contained some important principles of care, important especially as some have yet to be realised:
1. The institution should not be a stagnant pool but a flowing lake.
2. The object should be to prepare patients for life in the community, not simply to confine them for life.
3. The real criterion of mental deficiency should be social in-efficiency, not educational subnormality.
4. The establishment of the 'Half Way House'.
5. The institution should be more like a boarding school than a hospital.

Nearly fifty years later we have yet to make a significant move in this direction.

The Education Act of 1944 made special provision for the

8 COMMUNITY PSYCHIATRIC NURSING

educationally subnormal, yet unfortunately excluded from school the more severely handicapped:

During the 1950s through the work of the Clarkes (10) it became apparent that the mentally handicapped could learn if appropriately taught. The 1959 Mental Health Act placed the emphasis on community care and an absence of compulsion with the exception of that of attendance at a training centre under the auspices of the Health Service. This reflects the notion of the clinical nature of mental handicap rather than one of education.

The situation was remedied in 1971 with the Education (Handicapped Children) Act and centres became special schools with trained teachers. The adult training centres became the responsibility of the Social Services Department in the same year.

Despite the work of the Hospital Advisory Service the hospital service remained medically dominated providing inadequate or inappropriate care. On February 26th, 1975, Barbara Castle introduced a four point plan to improve the service:

1. National Development Group under the chairmanship of Peter Mittler.
2. National Development Team.
3. An inquiry into mental handicap nursing and care, chaired by Peggy Jay.
4. The role of the medical specialist to be reviewed.

Since that time the National Development Group have issued a number of bulletins, all of which should not only be read, but studied, and acted upon by the community nurse.

Of the role of the psychiatrist, little has been heard, which is not the case with the inquiry under the chairmanship of Peggy Jay, which belongs to the future and a later chapter.

REFERENCES

1. Walk, A. (1961) History of mental nursing, *The Journal of Mental Science*, No. 446, Vol. 107.
2. Clarke, B. (1975) *Mental Disorder in Earlier Britain*. Cardiff: University of Wales Press.
3. Skultans, V. (1975) *Madness and Morals*. London: Routledge and Kegan Paul.
4. Foucault, M. (1967) *Madness and Civilisation*. London: Tavistock Publications.
5. Jones, K. (1955) *Lunacy Law and Conscience 1744–1845*. London: Routledge and Kegan Paul.
6. Goddard, L. (1953) History of mental nursing, *The British Journal of Nursing*, June.
7. Greene, B. (1975) The rise and fall of the Asylum Workers' Association, *Nursing Mirror*, December 25th.
8. Mental Hospital and Institutional Workers' Union (1931) *A History of the Mental Hospital and Institutional Workers' Union 1910–1931*. Manchester: Express Co-operative Printing Co. Ltd.

9. H.M.S.O (1929) Report of the Mental Deficiency Committee. London.
10. Clarke, A. M. and Clarke, A. D. B. (1958) *Mental Deficiency* – The Changing Outlook. London: Methuen.

FURTHER READING

Deutsch, A. (1946) *The Mentally Ill in America*. New York: Colombia University Press.
Grob, G. N. (1973) *Mental Institutions in America*. New York: The Free Press.
Howells, J. C. (1975). *World History of Psychiatry*. London: Bailliere Tindall.

2

Ideology and mental health

It is, of course, important in any historical review to trace not only the deeds that were performed but also to look closely at the ideas that gave them birth.

The concept of 'ideology' is one which has increased in both use and importance over recent years. Fowler(1) describes it as follows:

> The modern vogue of the word 'ideology' is a natural result of the decline of religious faith. We have had to find a word, free from the religious association of 'faith' and 'creed', for belief in those politics—social systems vaguely indicated by such words as 'democracy', 'socialism', 'communism', and 'fascism', which excite in their adherents a quasi-religious enthusiasm. 'Ideology' (the science of ideas) lay ready to hand, the more acceptable because it seemed to suggest striving for an ideal. It was therefore pressed into this new service, which has now become its main occupation.

We tend accordingly to think of 'ideology' in terms of the political arena—'Communism' v 'Capitalism', or the 'Right' v the 'Left'. In fact, ideologies go far beyond that now, and are to be found in quite a number of other areas—the economic, the medical and legal professions, the religious sphere, and in the sexual and social arenas. As Brown(2) notes, ideologies are used to sustain differences not only between East and West and Right and Left, but also between black and white, rich and poor, young and old, and men and women.

The power and influence of ideologies is truly phenomenal—one has only to glance at a few of the names to recognise this: Moses, Christ, Machiavelli, Luther, Rousseau, Marx, Weber, Napoleon, Freud, Hitler, Gandhi, Mao Tse-Tung. Their influence long outlives them, and in fact often increases with time. The themes they preach, because of the simple but powerful message, are often associated with catch-phrases, epigrams, or slogans, more often than not written by others. Thus—to us in the West—the socialist states, of Eastern Europe particularly, are viewed in terms of George Orwell's 'big brother is watching you', while we in the West are looked upon as slaves to the capitalist ethic forever foraging away in some latter-day version of William Blake's 'dark satanic mills'. A recent classic was

Mao Tse-Tung's 'political power grows out of the barrel of a gun'. Such phrases are 'too sweet to be wholesome' intellectually, but they serve to reinforce the nature of the particular ideology.

Psychiatry is a discipline peculiarly susceptive to ideology. This may well stem from the intangible nature of its stock-in-trade—the mind and all its complexities. Four distinct ideologies have influenced psychiatric practice, some more dynamically than others, and we must now turn our attention to these.

Freud could be said to have been the first ideologue of psychiatry. As Szasz(3) puts it: '. . . psychiatry became (as a result of Freud's work) a popular ideology with "mental health and mental illness" its key symbols'. His influence pervaded not just psychiatry but society during the twentieth century. La Piere(4) puts it thus: 'It (the Freudian ethic) has become the ethic that is most commonly advocated by the intellectual leaders of the United States'. In the context of psychiatric practice, psychotherapy owes its origins to Freud's formulation of psychoanalysis, and his has been the dominant influence on the development of psychotherapeutic techniques. One of the more celebrated figures in psychotherapy today is, of course, R. D. Laing(5): 'All distinctions are mind, by mind, in mind, of mind. No distinctions no mind to distinguish'. North(6) contends as follows: 'The psychoanalytic movement in its various forms has had an impact on academic and popular thought that is probably only equalled by that of Marxism'.

If we move away from the introspective world of Freud and his followers and come to the mechanistic world of the behaviourists, we light upon our second influence on psychiatric thought and practice. Behaviourism was founded by J. B. Watson who was contemporaneous with Freud but who was deeply influenced by the work of Pavlov on the 'conditioned reflex'. Among its more famous exponents today are Skinner and Eysenck. Adherents of this school of thought reject Freud and his successors' emphasis on introspection—along with, incidentally, the 'functionalist' psychology of William James and the Gestalt psychology of Wertheiner and Kohler, and instead they advocate 'objectivity' through laboratory experiments with both animals and humans, and insist on treating symptoms rather than causes. As an ideology 'behaviourism' is pervasive today, and is one of the strongest single influences on psychology and sociology in this country at the moment. Goble (1970)(7) notes as follows:

Still more recently (1968), a distinguished panel of scholars, representing a first-hand knowledge of behavioural science trends in England, Europe, India, Africa and Australia, concluded that the trend in these countries was away from Freudianism towards behaviourism. (Sixth annual meeting of American Associates of Humanistic Psychology, August 27th–29th, 1968, San Francisco, California).

It is interesting to observe that exponents of behaviourism have never become ideologues or charismatic figures in the way that exponents of psychotherapy have. Perhaps the psychotherapists through their greater awareness of the 'inner man' are able to project their personalities and their ideas more ably than the behaviourists who seek only neutral objectivity. This may indeed help to explain why in a 'techno-tific' society, impersonal and increasingly valueless, the cult of behaviourism and its associated therapeutic tool, behaviour modification/therapy, have waxed strong.

'Third force psychology' is the name which Abraham Maslow gave to the new movement in psychology known as 'humanistic psychology', and also describes a third area of influence on psychiatry from the field of psychology. As Maslow himself was the first to admit (cf. Goble)(7) this new movement owes its origins to many—Carl Jung, Alfred Adler, Gordon Allport, and Carl Rogers, to mention but a few. The central tenets of this new approach are outlined as follows by Goble:

> a dissatisfaction with pathology-centred theories; a recognition of man's potential to grow and to determine his own future; a cognizance that man does not live by bread alone, but has common higher needs; an approach that considers man's feelings, desires, and emotions instead of examining him as one would a lump of coal; a recognition that there is such a thing as right and wrong which can be determined through observation and experience; the belief that responsibility is healthy and irresponsibility is costly.

This movement rejects, on the one hand Freud's 'dictatorship of the subconscious', and on the other, the objective experimentalist approach of the behaviourists which seems to look on man as a machine—a sum of all his parts. The 'humanists' see man as adding up to more than that—they place man, whole man, at the centre of things, and see him as one who determines rather than one who is determined by. This new approach has expressed itself in a variety of therapeutic ways. Rogers(8) lists them as follows:

T-group;

Encounter group;

Sensitivity training group;

Task-orientated group;

Sensory awareness groups, body awareness groups, body movement groups;

Creativity workshops;

Organisational development group;

Team building group;

Gestalt group;

Synanon group or 'game'.

The therapeutic tools generated by humanistic psychology have had less effect on psychiatric practice than either psychotherapy or behavioural therapy because, as Rogers notes, they are viewed with no small degree of suspicion by the establishment which has not yet absorbed them—Szasz, of course, believes that one of the main features of psychiatry is that it upholds the establishment. (David Cooper has said somewhere—perhaps in one of the 'Sunday glossies'—that one of the major triumphs of British psychiatry has been to absorb new ideas without in any way radically altering its practice!)

The fourth great ideology in the field of mental health is, of course, medicine. Medicine as an ideology is extremely old, dating back to classical Greece at least; medicine as an ideology in psychiatry is also old, dating back to the sixteenth century—Johann Weyer (1515–88) is regarded by many to have been the first psychiatrist. The process of integrating psychiatry with medicine has however been a lengthy one, and was probably not completed until after the last war. Martin(9) notes that since then psychiatry has been integrated within medicine to such an extent that it is now on an equal footing with the other specialist areas of practice. (The concrete evidence for this may be seen in the shape of the District General Hospital Psychiatric Unit, Carr(10). Despite its age, medicine as an ideology in psychiatry has been little studied and is therefore insufficiently understood. We know the components of the medical model—Siegler and Osmond(11) give a very amusing account of them as they would be observed by a Martian spy, viz. hospital, patient, doctor, examination, diagnosis, treatment, prognosis, with the paradigm being characterised by 'urgent matters dealt with at a fast pace'. Knowing the components is one thing—evaluating the place of medicine in psychiatry is another. Have we really got any further than the position reached when nineteenth-century psychiatry converged on Freud:

> Thus while the victim of mental illness is entirely alienated in the real person of his doctor, the doctor dissipates the reality of the mental illness in the critical concept of madness. So that there remains, beyond the empty forms of positivist thought, only a single concrete reality: the doctor–patient couple in which all alienations are summarised, linked, and loosened.   (Foucault)(12)

The trouble with ideologies is that their devotees and adherents tend to see their particular ideology as the only one, and they dismiss others as being inappropriate or worse. Thus, while doctors view the medical model with pride and delight, psychotherapists gaze starry-eyed at Freud and his successors; and whilst the neo-Freudian revisionists are busy at their work, the behaviourists are doggedly experimenting away certain that they will one day unscrabble the intricacies of human behaviour and thus reduce man to a set of responses. Nurses have always been at the beck and call of others, ideologically as well as every other way and this is no less true of mental or mental handicap nurses than it is of all other nurses. One could liken psychiatric nurses—to use a generic phrase to cover the above two groups—to so many grains of sand ceaselessly washed this way and that by successive tides of ideology, and when not awash, forever trodden on by others intent on playing out some particular therapy/treatment game. (It may be interesting to speculate that there is a causal link here: perhaps because nursing has always operated in an ideology-free context it has therefore put itself at the disposal of other ideologically-orientated practitioners. The lack of an ideology to a group of practitioners may be like a vacuum in the natural world—to be abhorred!)

We have looked at the ideologies which dynamically affected psychiatry from without—let us now turn our attention to how psychiatry withstood the external stresses and strain to which it was subjected and formulated from within philosophies which sustained its practitioners. Geertz(13) defines ideology related to the professional arena as follows: '... to render otherwise incomprehensible social situations meaningful, to so construe them as to make it possible to act purposefully within them'. Ideologies, then, in a professional sense, are belief systems which enable people to act in concert towards some particular end. Marx(14) suggests the following three criteria in relation to the generation of an ideology in any particular field of practice:

1. newness or rapid expansion;
2. a premium on a particularistic, subjective, or intuitive approach to the application of knowledge;
3. a moral or ethical aura surrounding the subject matter.

These criteria apply well to psychiatry, which may go some way in explaining why it has had more than its fair share of ideology. The differences are well-documented:

1. 'humanism versus custodialism'—Gilbert and Levinson(15) Sharaf and Levinson(16);
2. analytical and psychotherapeutic versus the directive—organic— Hollingshead and Redlich(17);
3. while Strauss et al.(18) described the contemporary ideologies as:
   a. psychotherapeutic ⎫
   b. somatotherapeutic ⎬ orientations
   c. sociotherapeutic ⎭

We see accordingly that the intra-professional ideologies very clearly mirror the inter-professional and all-encompassing behavioural, in the broadest sense, ideologies of the twentieth century, viz. Freudianism versus behaviourism with medicine increasingly acting as the framework around which new theories were constructed.

Even Strauss and his colleagues—in their notable work(18)—failed to take account of the 'community orientation' as an ideology—an ideology which would increasingly require professional roles to change and expand in the direction of assuming responsibility for those who needed help but were unable/unwilling to seek it. Their omission is surprising in the light of the fact that in the same year as they published, Bellak(19) hailed the community mental health movement as the 'third psychiatric revolution'. The movement had begun as a response to President Kennedy's call for a 'bold, new approach' to the care and treatment of the mentally ill, and was in every way a phenomenon fitted for the generation of an ideology, even right down to the slogans that accompanied it. In addition to Bellak's epigram above, Baker and Schulberg(20) describe community mental health as the 'belief system of the 1960s'. The same authors contend that their Community Mental Health Ideology Scale 'supports the hypothesis that there exists a relatively coherent belief system that differentially characterises today's mental health professionals'. Early studies in the U.S.A. with ideology scales did not look at psychiatric nurses as a professional group, and it was left to Howard and Baker(21) to remedy this deficiency. They found that graduate psychiatric nursing students showed a commitment to the ideas of community mental health which was greater than that shown by their professional colleagues—psychiatrists and psychologists—in the earlier studies. They conclude as follows:

> The community mental health ideology is viewed as posing a challenge to the development of nursing with an emphasis on a generalist rather than a specialist role; and as an opportunity to expand the development of nursing in the traditional path of doing whatever is necessary to improve the health status of the individual and the community.

So far as psychiatric nurses, to use the generic term once again, in this country are concerned, it is fairly safe to say that they have always operated, as suggested above, in an ideology-free context. Strauss *et al.*(18) have suggested that in institutions such as psychiatric hospitals it may be very difficult for nurses to do anything other than operate within the context of the prevailing medical ideology. The community however, offers an opportunity to nurses to break away from their traditional neutrality in relation to formulating an ideology, and to modify the medical model, which was probably the only model they were exposed to during training and subsequent practice, in the direction of humanising it. Much has been written of psychosocial nursing(22) and it may well be that an ideology appropriate for helping clients/patients/people will be formulated in the near future. That the time is now ripe for such an adventure cannot be doubted. A number of factors lead one to this conclusion.

First, we in the U.K. living as we do in a developed Western society are subject to the dominant prevailing ideology of industrialism. This, as Navarro(23) has pointed out, owes much to be writings of Max Weber(24) and is 'grounded largely in technological determinism'. The industrialised society makes other ideologies—christianity, capitalism, socialism—seem almost outmoded. Industrialism is viewed by differing theoreticians as good or bad—by an increasing number as the latter. Representing this group is Illich(25), who sees the institutions of society, including the medical bureaucracy, as arenas for conflict between the technocrats, i.e. those running the societal institutions, and the consumers of the goods and services administered by any particular bureaucratic organisation. The outcome of this conflict results in iatrogenesis—the consumer is harmed rather than helped by the bureaucracy. The approach, particularly of those who view the industrialised society as harmful has brought into focus the whole question of what health is/is not. Calls for the de-bureaucratisation and de-industrialisation of society in general and medicine in particular have been made in an attempt to slow down or even reverse the damage already done. The growth of community mental health as an ideology in the U.S.A. and the emergence of community psychiatric nursing in the U.K. are perhaps indications that a countervailing approach is in the process of formation.

Secondly, the stream of excellent reports emanating from the World Health Organisation(26) seem finally to have made an impression in the U.K. Recent official documents(27) all reflect the growing awareness of and concern with care in the community. Dr. David Owen, whilst Minister of Health, was most concerned in his recent book(28) to see 'concern for the mentally ill and handicapped' in terms of community provision. The community psychiatric nursing service is mentioned specifically—both mental illness and mental handicap branches—and greater use of the service is recommended by the then minister.

Thirdly, courses of training designed specifically for community psychiatric nurses—both mental handicap and mental nurses—now exist. Based on an 'outline syllabus' put out by the Joint Board of Clinical Nursing Studies (Course No. 800), these courses—running currently at Manchester Polytechnic, North East London Polytechnic, and The West London Institute of Higher Education—serve to bring together community psychiatric nurses for a whole academic year and thus create a forum for discussion which cannot but help in the formulation of an ideology appropriate for this new and expanding field of endeavour.

Fourthly, we have witnessed over the last couple of years the emergence and rapid growth of the Community Psychiatric Nurses' Association (C.P.N.A.). Now firmly established on a national footing, it operates through a regional network of officers and meetings. Local needs are thus identified and discussed at local level, and issues affecting community psychiatric nurses nationally are brought forward for national debate. Acting as both an educational and a professional body (it is in fact a registered charity), the Association brings together C.P.N.s in debate—a debate which will undoubtedly help in the process of establishing national values and consequently on all-embracing philosophy must eventually emerge.

Factors have been identified which indicate that an ideology for community psychiatric nursing may well be in the offing, but what kind of ideology will emerge? Ideology is undoubtedly important in the process of social change (cf. Levinson, and Tomkins(29))—an emergent philosophy must therefore at one and the same time reflect the colossal change that is taking place in society and serve as a guide in adapting the system to the changing needs of people in distress and society in 'future shock' (cf. Toffler(30)). The exact shape of such an ideology is uncertain at the moment—its image will not be brought sharply into focus until a number of fuzzy areas are resolved, notably those relating to structure of services, roles of practitioners, and the extent of future provision. Nevertheless, it is possible perhaps to delineate certain features which will characterise the community psychiatric nursing ideology:

it will be generalist in nature—C.P.N.s will encounter in their work the vast generality of people, and to operate within an ideological framework which adopted a particularist stance would preclude objective assessment and response;

it will be pluralistic in nature—C.P.N.s must be aware of the range of philosophies and their concomitant treatments in order to be able to respond, or provide a response through others, that is appropriate not to the principles of some particular treatment regime but rather to the special needs of the person/family in distress;

it will be person-centred—C.P.N.s are gradually moving out from under the shadow of the institution and will more and more come to see their function as one of helping people who are in need of their skills: they will make themselves, like St. Paul, 'all things to all men'.

18 COMMUNITY PSYCHIATRIC NURSING

REFERENCES

1. Fowler, H. W. (1965) *Modern English Usage.* Oxford: Oxford University Press.
2. Brown, C. B. (1973) *Ideology.* Harmondsworth: Penguin Books Ltd.
3. Szasz, T. S. (1974) *Ideology and Insanity.* Harmondsworth: Penguin Books Ltd.
4. La Piere, R. (1959) *The Freudian ethic.* New York: Duell, Sloan & Pierce.
5. Laing, R. D. (1970) *Knots.* London: Tavistock Publications Ltd.
6. North, M. (1975) *The Mind Market.* London: George Allen & Unwin Ltd.
7. Goble, F. G. (1970) *The Third Force.* New York: Grossman Publishers, Inc.
8. Rogers, C. R. (1969) *Encounter Groups.* Harmondsworth: Penguin Books Ltd.
9. Martin, D. V. (1968) *Adventure in Psychiatry.* Oxford: Bruno Cassirer.
10. Carr, P. J. 'To describe the role of the nurse working in a psychiatric unit which is situated in a district general hospital complex.' Unpublished Ph.D. Thesis, University of Manchester, 1979.
11. Siegler, M. and Osmond, H. (1974) *Models of Madness, Models of Medicine.* New York: Macmillan Publishing Co., Inc.
12. Foucault, M. (1967) *Madness and Civilisation.* London: Tavistock Publications Ltd.
13. Geertz, C. (1964) Ideology as a cultural system. In *Ideology and Dissent.* Apter, D. E. (ed.) New York: Free Press.
14. Marx, J. H. (1969) A multidimensional conception of ideologies in professional arenas: the case of the mental health field. *Pacific Sociological Review,* **12** (Fall), 75–85.
    N.B. I am indebted for the previous two references, and also for other material to an article by Wagenfeld, M. O., entitled The primary prevention of mental illness: A sociological perspective. In *Journal of Health and Social Behavior.* I am not able to uncover the exact references, but the article was probably published in 1971/72.
15. Gilbert, D. C. and Levinson, D. J. (1957) 'Custodialism' and 'humanism' in staff ideology. In *The patient and the Mental Hospital.* Greenblatt, M., Levinson, D. J. and Williams, R. H. (eds) Glencoe, Ill: The Free Press.
16. Sharaf, M. and Levinson, D. J. (1957) Patterns of ideology and role differentiation among psychiatric residents. In *The patient and the Mental Hospital.* Greenblatt, M., Levinson, D. J. and Williams, R. H. (eds) Glencoe, Ill: The Free Press.
17. Hollingshead, A. B. and Pedlich, F. C. (1958) *Social Class and Mental Illness.* New York: John Wiley and Sons.
18. Strauss, A., Schatzman, L., Bucher, R., Erlich, D. and Sabshin, H. (1964) *Psychiatric Ideologies and Institutions.* New York: The Free Press of Glencoe.
19. Bellak, L. (1964) *Community Psychiatry and Community Mental Health.* New York: Grune and Stratton.
20. Baker, F. and Schulberg, H. C. (1967) The development of a community mental health ideology scale, *Community Mental Health Journal,* **3,** 216–225.
21. Howard, L. A. and Baker, F. (1971) Ideology and role function of the nurse in community mental health, *Nursing Research,* **20,** 450–454.
22.
a. Evans, F. M. C. (1971) *Psychosocial Nursing: Theory and Practice in Hospitals and Community Mental Health.* New York: Macmillan Publishing Co., Inc.
b. Chapman, A. H. and Almeida, E. M. (1972) *The Interpersonal Basis of Psychiatric Nursing.* New York: Putman.
c. Robinson, L. (1972) *Psychiatric Nursing as a Human Experience.* Philadelphia: Saunders.
d. Marram, C. D. (1973) *The Group Approach to Nursing Practice.* St. Louis: The C. V. Mosby Co.
e. Loomis, M. E. and Horsley, J. A. (1974) *Interpersonal Change: A Behavioural Approach to Nursing Practice.* New York: McGraw-Hill.

f.   Smoyak, S. (ed.) (1975) *The Psychiatric Nurse as a Family Therapist*. New York: Wiley.

g.   Towell, D. (1975) *Understanding Psychiatric Nursing*. London: Royal College of Nursing.

23.   Navarro, V. (1976) *Medicine under Capitalism*. New York: Prodist.

24.   Max Weber (1864-1920), was one of the founding fathers of sociology. He wrote extensively in such different areas as methodology, economic history, religion, and, of course, sociology. He foresaw the rise of bureaucracies—the rational institution—and regarded them with deep misgivings in relation to personal freedom and human values. Apart from his interest in 'rationality' *vis-a-vis* science and social science—the so-called 'value-free sociology—Weber was also fascinated by the religious spectrum in societies. Gouldner says of him: 'I have therefore come to believe that the value-free doctrine is, from Weber's standpoint, basically an effort to compromise two of the deepest traditions of Western thought, reason and faith, but that his arbitration seeks above all to safeguard the romantic residual in modern man.' (Gouldner, A. W. (1975) *For Sociology*. Harmondsworth Penguin Books Ltd.). Weber's notion of 'charisma' bears witness to Gouldner's conclusion. All Weber's books are now classics of sociology—some of them are landmarks in the history of social science:
The Theory of Social and Economic Organisation. New York: Free Press of Glencoe (1964);
The Protestant Ethic and the Spirit of Capitalism. New York: Scribner (1958). This last book, which left a profound impression on the social sciences, taken in conjunction with his works on the Jewish, Chinese, and Indian religions, betrayed the depth of his interest in this aspect of social behaviour—an interest shared incidentally by his contemporary, and one of the other founding fathers of sociology, Emile Durkheim. Weber was critical of Marx in his advocacy of the socialist economy, because he believed that such economies would be more bureaucratic than capitalist economies; and in any case, he was opposed to 'historical materialism'. Weber's influence is pervasive in sociology today, not least because the theory of social action—a foundation for sociology—has its roots in him. (Cf. Parsons, T., *The Structure of Social Action*. New York: Free Press of Glencoe).

25.   Illich, I. (1975) *Medical nemesis: the Expropriation of Health*. London: Calder and Boyers.

26.

a.   World Health Organisation (1956) *Expert Committee on Psychiatric Nursing—First Report*. Geneva: Technical Report Series 105.

b.   World Health Organisation (1959) *Seminar on the Nurse in the Psychiatric Team*. Noordwijk, 4–15 November, 1957. Copenhagen.

c.   World Health Organisation (1971) *Trends in Psychiatric Care: Day Hospitals and Units in General Hospitals*. Salzburg, June 7th–11th, 1971. Copenhagen.

d.   World Health Organisation (1974) *Evaluation of Mental Health Education Programmes: Report of a Working Group*. Nancy, May 21st–24th, 1973. Copenhagen.

27.

a.   *Better Services for the Mentally Handicapped*, Cmnd. 4683, HMSO. London, 1971.

b.   *Better Services for the Mentally Ill*, Cmnd. 6233, HMSO, London, 1975.

c.   Department of Health and Social Security, *Priorities for Health and Personal Social Services in England*, a Consultative Document, HMSO, London, 1976.

28.   Owen, D. (1976) *In Sickness and in Health*. London: Quartet Books.

29.

a.   Levinson, D. J. (1964) Idea systems in the individual and society. In *Explorations in Social Change*. Zollscham, G. K. and Hirsch, W. (eds) Boston: Houghton Mifflin.

b. Tomkins, S. S. (1965) Affect and the psychology of knowledge. In *Affect, Cognition, and Personality*. Tomkins, S. S. and Izard, C. E. (eds) New York: Springer Publishing Co.

30. Toffler, A. (1971) *Future Shock*. London: Pan Books Ltd.

3

The emergence and development of the community psychiatric nursing team

From ideological paradigms to the developmental patterns of community psychiatric nursing services is perhaps not an easy stride, but in making it, the reader will see the indications which are already marking the route to a recognisable philosophical identity for community psychiatric nursing services in Great Britain.

One of the most interesting aspects of this development is that where services have proved the most startlingly successful is where they have established themselves counter to established psychiatric practice. Also the majority of services have been established despite considerable opposition from medical bureaucracy. The nursing profession has had to ride out some uncomfortable times in justifying the establishment of community psychiatric nursing services. In the end it appears that common sense has prevailed and if existing service were to be threatened, previously dedicated opponents would no doubt support the community psychiatric nursing cause.

Looking at the developmental progress of community psychiatric nursing provides an overview of the variety of types of service which have materialised as a response to local demands. Such a 'free thinking' approach by nurse managers who are at present unfettered by hierarchical edicts would not have produced such a variety of successes had the emphasis been on supplying a National Health Service blanket service. Community psychiatric nurses have benefited from the setting up of systems which 'supply psychiatric nursing needs' to the community rather than a defined service with stated boundaries. Like all new ideas however, there will eventually be some form of rationalisation, as there are inherent dangers in the letting loose of yet another service upon the community.

An interesting parallel is drawn by Kane(1):

> Professionals are staking claims in promising new territory and only later digging the theoretical mines necessary to determine whether they have struck an appropriate task

The services which exist at the moment have fundamental differences which can be put as simply as hospital base versus primary care team base, and secondly, referrals from hospital medical staff and ward staff versus and 'open' referral system which will advise and help anyone who expresses a need.

There are needs in all these areas and, hopefully, teams will eventually cover all the areas previously mentioned, as a restriction to narrow concepts only cuts down on a service which could and should be provided.

A closer examination of the development of community psychiatric nursing shows where different philosophies have led to different services and how the enormous growth in community psychiatric nursing services has taken place in the first half of the 1970's.

THE EMERGENCE AND PRESENT DAY ORGANISATION OF THE COMMUNITY PSYCHIATRIC NURSING SERVICES

Two of the earliest published papers to give a descriptive account of Community Psychiatric Nursing Services are those of

May A. R. and Moore S.(2) and Greene J.(3).

May and Moore describe the service which started at Warlingham Park Hospital in 1954. The service was organised for two main reasons:
1. Shortage of P.S.W.s.
2. Because of the recognition of a need for the continued supervision of patients following discharge.

Nurses were seconded to the Croydon borough and worked from a mental health centre attached to a day hospital. May and Moore go on to describe the underlying principles upon which the service was based.

> 1. Although the nurses are in contact with P.S.W.s, M.W.O.s and other local authority agents and though the greater part of their work lies outside the hospital, they should remain on the nursing establishment of the hospital and within its medico-nursing administrative framework.
> 2. Because of his/her training the qualified mental nurse is well fitted to assess the mental state of a patient, especially if he/she already knows the patient. It is in this nurse-patient relationship that the value of the out-patient nurse is most clearly seen.
> 3. The out-patient nurse* can reassure and encourage patients, supervise the medication prescribed by the doctor, detect defiencies in personal habits and care, and often remedy them and relieve the anxieties of relatives by timely explanation.

It is interesting to note that guidelines were already being set for the siting of the community psychiatric nursing service, its lines of responsibility and a broad outline of the role had been given, which

---

* out-patient nurse is the original title used to describe their community psychiatric nurses.

included medication supervision, family support and personal support through the nurse-patient relationship.

Greene(3) described a service which had been organised at Moorhaven hospital in 1957. This service used nurses who were working in the hospital setting thus giving them a dual role of hospital/community nurse. This service was also started because of a shortage of social work help and as Greene also states 'There remained a group of patients who needed the kind of attention that only psychiatric nurses could supply.'

Some ideas were emerging that nurses were not just filling spaces left by the shortage of social workers but that they also had a special service to offer the psychiatric patient in the community. Greene also goes on to summarise the nursing activities involved:

> a. To provide psychiatric nursing care of a physical or psychological nature in accordance with the doctors wishes for patients who have been discharged from hospital and who are in need of continuing nursing care.
> b. Working in close liaison with doctors and social workers as professional members of a therapeutic team.
> c. Extending to the patient and his family such support as may be reasonably regarded as part of a nurse's work.
> d. A preventive role in going to the aid of patients whose illness does not require treatment in a clinic or hospital.
> e. Being available in a consultative capacity to non-psychiatric nurses who may have problems with patients showing symptoms of nervous and mental disorders.

Both stated that the community psychiatric nurse had something special to offer, in the way of nursing and were not 'substitute social workers'. From 1969 onwards there was a large increase in the number of community psychiatric nursing services throughout the country. The reasons for this are varied. There is no doubt that the changing awareness of the potential role of the psychiatric nurse played a major part in this rise and more recently the re-organisation of the social services had its impact on the services provided to the mentally ill and handicapped in the community. This is looked at in some detail by Hunter(4) in his comprehensive review of the rise of community psychiatric nursing in Britain. It can be argued that the community psychiatric nursing service has now lost its 'nursing component'. Various authors have sought to establish a differential role between the social worker and the community psychiatric nurse. Most literature would agree that there are considerable 'grey' areas between the community psychiatric nurse and the social worker roles, as indeed exist between the community psychiatric nurse and the health visitor and most other para-medical and medical professionals. This role diffusion is inevitable and important but there does remain a special role for each professional.

Bennet(5) and Harris(6) have sought to establish the differences between the nursing and social needs of a patient following discharge from hospital. Altschul(7) goes to some lengths to point out the confusion which exists between the roles of various professionals in the community. In her description of the services in operation at Dingleton Hospital in Scotland she states:

> Evidence for differential use of professional skills was not produced, on the contrary (the use of check lists) confirmed that the culture of Dingleton which emphasised similarities in function, overlap of roles, role blurring and absence of role specificity was accepted by staff members who worked in the community.

This active move to blur role boundaries is probably not unique to Dingleton but it is not seen to such a great extent elsewhere. Barker(8) has described the role of the community psychiatric nurse as having four main areas and he describes 'The nurse assessor, the nurse consultant, the nurse therapist and the nurse clinician'. These four areas form a useful framework on which to base an outline of the role of the community psychiatric nurse and with the addition of the two other areas of the nurse educator and the nurse manager, some idea of the role of the community psychiatric nurse emerges.

The community psychiatric nurse as a consultant
Psychiatric nursing care is a resource which can be made available to the mentally disordered in the community. The community psychiatric nurse can give advice to other professionals in the community about the type and level of psychiatric nursing care required at any given time.

The community psychiatric nurse as a clinician
This is the nursing action undertaken in the care process it can be technical i.e. giving injections etc., or basic, such as ensuring the maintenance of an adequate diet.

The community psychiatric nurse as a therapist
Psychiatric nurses are now commonly involved in the therapeutic activities of psychotherapy and behaviouralism. The transfer of these treatments to the community is an essential part of the community psychiatric nurses' role and makes these treatments more accessible and realistic.

The community psychiatric nurse as an assessor
Assessment forms a vital part of any care giving service, community

psychiatric nurses can assess the nursing requirements of potential patients and having delivered that care, assess its effectiveness.

The community psychiatric nurse as an educator
The community psychiatric nurse has a responsibility to the community to educate people about the potential hazards of mental disorder. This education is not confined to the curative aspects but more importantly the preventive aspects. The education of other professions and nursing students is also an important factor.

The community psychiatric nurse as a manager
The complexities of communication in the community setting and the organisation of work priorities demands that the community psychiatric nurse be a competent manager.

These six areas encompass most of the component parts of the role of the community psychiatric nurse and most present day community psychiatric nurses are involved in all the mentioned areas. It is true that diversification into specialism has already occurred in some teams and some community psychiatric nurses already concentrate in such areas as behavioural techniques or alcoholism treatments. It is important to achieve the overall aims of a community psychiatric nursing service which should be the comprehensive delivery of psychiatric nursing skills to the community, before this specialisation is realised.

Official documentation which favours the development of community psychiatric nursing is a little thin on the ground but has been forthcoming in small quantities since the early 1970s. The General Nursing Council had recognised the fact that community experience is essential to student training in psychiatric/mental handicap nurse training. The two circulars 72/8/24 and 72/8/25 both point out the need. The World Health Organisation has also made a number of references to the importance of the psychiatric nurse in the community. In a later report the W.H.O. states:

> Since most psychiatric services are still confined to Hospitals and similar institutions, the bulk of nursing personnel are to be found in these settings. The need to extend psychiatric nursing care into the community health services outside these institutions was considered to be of primary importance.

The same report goes on to say:

> Emphasis in all mental health care nursing services should be placed on prevention and early detection of individuals and families of visit(10).

In this country the D.H.S.S. in its report(11) states:

The (health) district (psychiatric) nursing service in the new pattern will be responsible for meeting all the psychiatric nursing needs of mentally ill people from the district—whether as in-patients, out-patients or day-patients.
It will include community psychiatric nursing for patients living at home and specialist nursing advice to primary care teams.

A role for the community psychiatric nurse can now be identified and some official documentation is in support, but no guidelines exist to help the manager to decide on the site of community psychiatric nursing team or the methods of its functioning. All such information has been gathered by experience. Many services have been organised by juggling existing staffing establishments which are based on an institutional idea of staff to patient ratios. This makes estimation of required numbers difficult and the movement of staff harder to achieve.

In 1966, a report to the Royal College of Nursing was undertaken into the role of the psychiatric nurse in the community and some of the information received showed the following:

42 hospitals used nursing staff for community work.
35 hospitals used nursing staff for follow up work.
22 hospitals used nursing staff for drug supervision.
12 hospitals used nursing staff for injections.
26 nurses were used on a full-time basis and
220 were used on a part-time basis.

In 1974, J. W. Parnell wrote in the *Queen's Nursing Journal* that of the 15 regions all have a service in operation and of the 96 areas with 200 districts 150 services are in operation.

More localised surveys have taken place. In 1977 such a survey was undertaken by Shore(12) of the north-west region. The north-west region can be taken as being fairly representative for sample purposes. There are large areas of urban, rural and high density populations, it includes some nine single district areas one six district area and one three district area. They are obviously subject to the same regional influences (if as such it exists) on the development of community psychiatric nursing.

Table 1 Numbers of staff working in community nursing departments in the north-west region

	Full-time	Part-time
Nursing officers	17	–
Sisters/charge nurses	58	9
Staff nurses	1	0
S.E.N.'s	8	3
Nursing assistants	0	0

Shore asked a number of interesting questions during his interview/questionnaire and some of these are reproduced here.

Table 2 Question: What activities are community psychiatric nurses regularly involved in?

Area or district	1	2	3	4	5	6	7	8	9	10	11	12	13	14	15	16	17	Percentage Involvement
Age of service (years)	5	4	4	4	2	3	1	1	4	6	4	1	3	4	5	4	5	
Crisis intervention	1	1	1	1	1	1	1	1	1	1	1	1	0	1	1	1	1	94
Ward rounds	0	1	0	0	1	1	0	1	1	1	1	1	0	1	0	0	1	59
Clubs and social activities	1	1	1	0	1	0	0	1	1	1	1	0	1	1	1	0	0	65
Group work	0	1	0	0	0	0	0	0	1	1	0	0	0	0	0	0	0	18
Behaviour modification programmes	1	1	1	1	0	0	0	1	0	1	1	0	0	1	1	0	1	59
Domiciliary visits with consultants	1	1	1	0	1	0	1	1	1	1	1	1	1	1	1	1	1	88
Clinic sessions in health centres	0	1	0	1	0	1	0	1	1	1	1	1	1	0	0	0	1	59
1st referrals unaccompanied	0	1	1	1	1	1	0	1	1	1	1	0	1	1	1	1	1	82

1=involved regularly   0=rarely or not at all

First referrals unaccompanied refers to visits made by community psychiatric nurse to patients where the G.P. has requested a Domiciliary visit by the consultant psychiatrist and the aforesaid visits have been made prior to that of the consultant.

Table 3 Question: Do community psychiatric nurses liaise closely with other disciplines?

Area or district	1	2	3	4	5	6	7	8	9	10	11	12	13	14	15	16	17	18
Social workers	1	0	1	1	1	1	1	1	1	1	1	1	1	1	1	1	1	1
District nurses	1	1	0	0	1	1	1	1	1	1	1	1	1	1	1	1	1	X
Health visitors	1	1	0	1	1	1	1	1	1	1	1	1	1	1	1	1	1	X
General practitioners	1	1	0	1	1	1	0	1	1	1	1	1	1	0	1	1	1	X
Psychiatric nurses	1	1	1	1	1	1	0	1	1	1	1	1	1	1	1	1	1	1
Police	0	0	X	X	X	1	0	1	0	0	1	1	1	X	1	0	X	X
Clergy	0	0	X	0	X	X	0	1	0	0	1	0	0	1	1	1	1	X
Voluntary bodies	0	0	X	1	X	X	0	1	0	1	1	1	1	1	1	1	1	X
Probation officers	0	0	0	X	X	1	0	1	0	0	1	1	1	1	1	1	1	X
Others	0	0	X	X	X	X	1	1	0	1	1	0	1	1	1	0	0	X

1 = liaises closely.   X = liaises when necessary.   0 = does not liaise

Where six of the seven that closely liaise with 'others', 'others' refers to the psychologist and one of the disablement resettlement officers.

Table 4 Question: What is the average case load per nurse?

Area	1	2	3	4	5	6	7	8	9	10	11	12	13	14	15	16	17
Case load per nurse	71	45	35	45	35	35	84	50	45	130*	38	33	39	40	45	65	45

*This figure includes 35 patients who were looked upon as having priority.

If one includes the figure of 130 the average case load per nurse for the region works out at 52. If one accepts the figure of 35 an average of 45 emerges.

Table 5 Question: What is the source of the referrals in your area?

Area or district	1	2	3	4	5	6	7	8	9	10	11	12	13	14	15	16	17
Consultants	1	1	1	1	1	1	1	1	1	1	1	1	1	1	1	1	1
General practitioners	1	1	0	0	1	0	0	1	1	1	1	0	1	0	0	1	1
Primary health care team (ex G.P.'s)	1	1	0	1	1	0	0	1	1	0	1	0	1	0	0	1	0
Social workers	1	1	0	0	1	0	0	1	1	0	1	0	1	0	0	1	0
Para medical services	0	0	0	0	1	0	0	1	1	0	1	0	1	0	0	1	0
Other	0	0	0	0	0	0	0	0	1	0	1	0	1	0	0	1	0

1 = referrals accepted from   0 = referrals not accepted from

This survey shows the differences between the various areas in terms of miles done, case load numbers and establishment numbers and methods of operation. How is it possible to estimate the numbers of community psychiatric nurses needed and how can the best be achieved?

A number of bases could, theoretically, be used to estimate the number of community psychiatric nurses needed to service a given population figure. In the report Cmnd. 6233(11) the following is stated:

> In the light of present and expected future numbers of psychiatric nurses the D.H.S.S. is aiming at an initial target in each Health District if a level of psychiatric nurse staffing of 85 nurses per 100 000 population increasing gradually as resources permit to 100 nurses per 100 000 population. The present national average is in excess of 90 per 100 000 but they are not evenly distributed. There has not yet been enough experience of the working of the proposed pattern of services for the mentally ill and units for the elderly severely mentally ill, to issue mere detailed guidance of nurse staffing levels at this stage. In addition nurses will be needed to staff the psychiatric services for children and adolescents as well as other special units such as the regional security units.

This gives some idea about the future foundations upon which all psychiatric nurse staffing levels are to be based. The present ratio of one nurse to three in patients should have been accomplished in all mental illness hospitals and although possible satisfying the institutions' needs does not provide a working model for a community service.

What base can be used to define the work load of community psychiatric nurses? Methods of operation vary so much from one team to another it is not possible to define a common method of referral or identify a referral source. Some services operate an 'open' referral system which means accepting referrals from all community workers such as health visitors, district nurses and general practitioners. Others limit their service to consultant psychiatrists and hospital based staff. If we examine both types of service and look at the referral

Table 6 A more detailed picture of the survey result is outlined here

Area Dist.	Catch. pop. '000s	Geog. Desc.	ATTA	Age of service	Establishment numbers initially	Establishment numbers at present	Nurses with C.P.N. cert.	Case load per nurse	Miles per mth. per nurse	Miles per mth. serv. total	Mthly visits per service	Total 1976	Visits 1st year	Patients seen at base 1967	Patients seen at base year 1	New refs per month 1976	New refs per month year 1
1	320	50/50	M	5	6	16	0	71	800	12800	1169	14034	N/A	150	N/A	35	N/A
2	280	MU	G	4	2	4	1	45	400	1600	246	2957	N/A	0	0	27	N/A
3	270	50/50	C	4	1	3	1	35	600	1800	N/A	N/A	N/A	N/A	N/A	N/A	N/A
4	313	MU	G	4	2	4	0	45	700	2800	400	4800	N/A	0	0	40	N/A
5	279	MU	C	2	2	2	0	35	500	1000	186	2240	N/A	0	0	N/A	N/A
6	312	MU	C	3	1	8	0	35	800	6400	833	10000	5500**	0	0	50	N/A
7	200	50/50	C	1	1	1	0	84	1000	1000	N/A	N/A	N/A	N/A	N/A	N/A	N/A
8	120	TU	M	1	1	3	0	50	500	1500	N/A	N/A	N/A	att HC	N/A	70	N/A
9	370	MU	M	4	4	7	0	45	900	6300	708	8500	N/A	3000	N/A	70	N/A
10	252	50/50	M	6	1	3	0	130	300	900	N/A	N/A	N/A	N/A	N/A	N/A	N/A
11	250	MU	G	4	1	3	0	38	400	1200	N/A	N/A	N/A	N/A	N/A	N/A	N/A
12	170	50/50	GP	1	2	2	0	33	350	700	67	N/A	335	N/A	5	N/A	5
13	180	MU	C	3	1	2	1	39	650	1300	N/A	N/A	2001	N/A	N/A	77	N/A
14	300	TU	C	4	2	4	0	40	500	2000	315	3784	N/A	0	0	12	N/A
15	111	MU	M	5	2	6	0	45	950	5700	589	7068	N/A	0	0	N/A	N/A
16	274	Mu	G	4	2	6	0	65	600	3600	N/A	N/A	N/A	N/A	N/A	N/A	N/A
17	200	TU	C	5	2	6	1	45	900	3600	600	7200	1300	0	0	50	N/A
18	158	MU	C	3	2	2	2	N/A	200	400	80	764	31	N/A	N/A	N/A	N/A

MU – Mostly Urban
TU – Totally Urban
50/50 – Mixture of Urban and Rural

M – Mixed
C – Consultant
G – Geographically
GP – General Practitioner

N/A – Not Available

* – Community Based
** – second year

rates it is possible to identify the sort of numbers that a service offering their expertise to both people in hospital and the community could expect to deal with.

Type A
Services which accept referrals only from consultants and hospital staff.

Service 1	*Mixed urban and rural*	
	Referrals for one year	423
	Number of community psychiatric nurses	2
	Population served	270 000
Service 2	*Totally urban*	
	Referrals for one year	588
	Number of community psychiatric nurses	3
	Population served	250 000
Service 3	*Mixed urban and Rural*	
	Referrals for one year	634
	Number of community psychiatric nurses	3
	Population served	270 000
Service 4	*Totally urban*	
	Referrals for one year	542
	Number of community psychiatric nurses	3
	Population served	250 000

There are an average of 199 referrals to each community psychiatric nurse from the hospital service in any one year. It must be remembered that these are new referrals and this will not take account of existing case loads.

Type B
Services which accept an open referral system from all community personnel, therefore, these patients have not been seen by a hospital or psychiatrist before.

Team 1	*Mixed urban and rural*	
	Referrals for one year	211
	Number of community psychiatric nurses	2
	Population served	282 000
Team 2	*Totally urban*	
	Referrals for one year	268
	Number of community psychiatric nurses	2
	Population served	280 000
Team 3	*Mixed Urban and Rural*	
	Referrals for one year	197

Number of community psychiatric nurses	2
Population served	170 000

Team 4   *Totally urban*

Referrals for one year	286
Number of community psychiatric nurses	3
Population served	250 000

There is an average of 106 referrals to each community psychiatric nurse and again this does not take into account existing case loads.

This is a very rudimentary way of examining the case loads and referral rate. The only way to do this with any degree of accuracy is to examine the prevalence of mental illness in the community. This method effectively covers both the people seen in hospital and both the psychiatric services and those who are going to stay within the community and do not need hospital services.

For a most comprehensive breakdown of projected figures for inception and incidence rates of mental illness in the community, Hicks(13) has collected together a number of surveys taken over a period of 30 years. His survey provides a remarkable insight into the dynamics of referral, consultation and incidence of mental disorder at the level of primary care. Hicks makes points of considerable interest to community psychiatric nurses.

> None of the doctors (in the survey) wished to get rid of or avoid the burden of dealing with their psychiatrically ill patients. The treatment that was attempted was often haphazard and inadequate and this was as unsatisfactory to the doctors as to the patients.

(Paragraph 885 as above)

Again, Shepherd *et al.*(14) give some idea of the treatment and management of psychiatric patients by diagnostic category. Some interesting facts emerge: only 9.1 per cent of all such patients seen were referred to a psychiatrist or for mental hospital admission, and only 4.8 per cent of the neurotic patients seen in the study were referred in this way.

Therefore, it is better to base the number of community psychiatric nurses required not on numbers referred from hospital consultants but, as is much more realistic, on populations statistics and the incidence of mental disorder in that community.

Watts, in a review of data from the morbidity study(15) puts the consulting rate at a mean of 50 per 1000 (around a range of 18–208). There is, however, some evidence of variance in reporting of some disorders in the study.

More recently, in a survey by Shepherd *et al.*(14) the authors report an annual prevalence rate (the number of patients consulting with psychiatric illness per 1000 at risk) at 140 per 1000. They place the inception rate for the population (new illness consulting during one year) at 52 per 1000.

A decision has then to be made about how many of these patients would or could be referred to a community psychiatric nurse. Driver(16), in her research in the Chester area in which she interviewed a number of general practitioners, found that they estimated 30.5 per cent of their patients had a mental illness component in their presenting complaint. Driver goes on to say:

> The statistics for the Chester District to April 1st, 1976 state the average number of patients per practice is 2399. Therefore each General Practitioner has approximately 732 patients who would fit into the above mentioned category and of these patients the General Practitioners interviewed said they would like to refer on average 13.13 per cent or 96 patients to a community psychiatric nursing service were it more freely available.

A working plan of the preceding figures looks like this:

1. One community psychiatric nurse per 15 000 population
Psychiatric illness incidence per population

Therefore in 15 000 = 140 per 1000 (Shepherd *et al*) = 2100
Patients to be referred to community psychiatric nurse
= 13.13% (Driver)
This is equal to 275.73 patients per C.P.N.

2. One community psychiatric nurse per 7500 population
This is equal to 137.86 patients per community psychiatric nurse.

The figure given at (1) appears more realistic than those given at (2) but it must be borne in mind that not all patients will be kept on a long term basis by the community psychiatric nurse and many of the patients will be a shared responsibility and kept on a 'one off' consultation basis. There is one additional fact of administrative loading which was set to health visitors at 5 per cent (Jamison Report, 1956). It would therefore appear that one community psychiatric nurse per 15 000 population is a feasible figure to aim for in the short term and half this figure in years to come would not be unreasonable.

This is only a basic guide and evidently only the tip of the iceberg. The psychiatric services can expect an increasing load from the elderly. Leopoldt (17) describes the attempt by an Oxford Service to deal with this problem and states:

> Although 50 per cent of the in-patient population of pscyhiatric hospitals falls into the over 65 age group only 5 per cent of the elderly in the community enter institutions for long term permanent care. The accumulated psychiatric, medical and nursing skills, as yet almost

exclusively concentrated in psychogeriatric hospital units, have to be spread more widely and evenly by various means into the community.

As Leopoldt also states 'In 1940 the rate of over 65s was one in twelve in 1970 it was one in six' and also 'concerning psychiatric morbidity in the elderly at least $1/5$ of people over 60 suffer from some form of mental disorder.'

This increasingly large group of people will have to be accounted for when services are to be organised to cater for future needs. It is obvious that a lot of research must be done into this area.

EVALUATION OF COMMUNITY PSYCHIATRIC NURSING SERVICE EFFECTIVENESS

If so many psychiatric nurses are moving out into the community, what is the result of this move, and how can services measure the effects of their work?

To evaluate the services offered by a community psychiatric nursing team cannot just be measured in terms of keeping 'x' number of patients out of hospital. This is an essential part of preventive psychiatric nursing but other effects need to be measured, e.g. effects on the family, effects on the community, effects on the patient and the cost effectiveness of a community psychiatric nursing team.

Community psychiatric nursing services have a number of goals which need to be measured to ascertain their effectiveness. These can be identified as follows:

Reduction of hospitalisation and the onset of mental illness
By the effective use of primary and secondary preventive nursing one of the main goals should be the prevention of the onset of mental illness. To measure this effectively is difficult. Some areas now have the benefit of a case register. Registers such as this can identify basic personal and clinical data for each individual patient and records the services they have received and the effect on that particular individual can be traced. This would only be applicable in the case of secondary prevention, primary preventive treatment is much more difficult to measure. Community surveys would be, perhaps, the only way to measure the effect of a service in this area, at the moment such surveys are not available and beyond the financial scope of the D.H.S.S. Where registers do exist the results have been documented (18, 19, 20). Registers may help structured community psychiatric nursing development in the future.

Effects on the family of community psychiatric nursing services

When a community psychiatric nursing service deals with any patient it will inevitably have some effect on the family as well. In an interesting paper Sainsbury (21) points to the types of behaviour which families of the mentally ill found to be the most troublesome.

Table 7

Behaviour	Percentage of families (410 patients)
Frequent complaints about bodily symptoms	38
A danger to himself (suicide/accident)	34
Importunate and demanding	34
Behaving oddly or expressing peculiar ideas	27
Unco-operative and contrary	26
Constantly restless or over-talkative by day	23
Troublesome at night	21
Threatening the safety of others	12
Objectionable, rude or embarrassing	8
Causing trouble with neighbours	7

Sainsbury also says 'the demented elderly and the psychopathic personalities were the two groups that taxed their families most.'

Using a more conventional control group and a community orientated psychiatric service, families of patients were followed up for two years and Sainsbury states 'all measures showed the community service left families more heavily burdened.'

But of particular importance was the finding that the mental health of the closest relative was significantly more affected in the community orientated service 'an observation which obliges us to consider whether the cost of keeping certain patients at home will be more illness in the community.'

This is a point of view once re-enforced by Kessel (22) who described community care services as 'the management of the patient in the community for as long as possible despite the difficulties this caused to the patients, their relatives and their general practitioners.'

These aspects of the effects of a community psychiatric nursing service will at some time need to be measured. The goal of such a service should be to relieve the pressure of the families of the mentally ill as well as to help the patient. A study of the effects of community psychiatric nurse intervention would be of interest. The studies mentioned perhaps serves as a caution to the current enthusiasm for community based treatment without adequate preparation of relatives and staff involved.

Cost effectiveness of community psychiatric nursing services

It requires very little mathematics to demonstrate the cost effectiveness of keeping 20 patients at home rather than in a ward setting. If these people are back at home working and being visited by a community psychiatric nurse once a week then this is sound economics. If these 20 people are all drawing social security, claiming rent rebates and other assorted benefits, then the economics of community care becomes less attractive.

Even in this setting however, the therapeutic benefits probably compensate for the narrowed margin of cost benefit. Warren (23) has made an attempt at evaluating the cost of ward staff visiting patients now discharged to the community for injection purposes and the cost of these patients were they now staying in hospital. He shows that this makes sound economics but goes on to say:

> However, it is difficult to assess in money the result of a physical assault by a mentally disturbed husband on his wife, the clamour of the neighbours demanding action from the police for an abusive woman in their midst, the squalor and filth of a neglected house or the effect on young children living in a disturbed home.

True cost effectiveness needs to be measured in these terms which is an impossible task. Some costs can be measured e.g. drug and equipment expenditure, mileage allowances and running costs, as they become better known community psychiatric nursing services will be asked to give account of their expenditure, and at the same time their justification in terms of money.

Siting of a community psychiatric nursing service

From the inception of community psychiatric nursing services there has been considerable discussion as to the most suitable site for such a service. Should teams be based in hospital, community or health centres, or a mixture of the three? Decisions have also had to be made about the way in which a service should be attached to medical staff (if at all) and whether or not a geographical responsibility is required by each nurse.

The value of forward planning and open consultation between all interested parties can pay dividends in the long term when setting up community psychiatric nursing services. White (24) describes the co-operation achieved between hospital and local authority when setting up a service in Buckinghamshire. There are a great number of articles which describe the end results of setting up a service in its various forms. Greene (2) and May and Moore (3) being amongst the first and then followed by a large number of descriptive articles (25, 26, 27, 28).

There is no doubt that most differences between community

psychiatric nursing services have arisen out of a need to meet local demands. What proves to be an ideal service for a densely populated urban area will not prove to be the right service for a large rural catchment area. Where ever services are operating they need to bear in mind some of the following points:

Planning to meet the needs of the community

One of the questions which must be asked is whether the service intends to serve the needs of the hospital or serve the needs of the community. Such items as geographical attachment need to be examined. This does not always coincide with consultant attachment in the hospital setting. In some cases one must be sacrificed for the other. In terms of local knowledge, economy and ease of access then geographical attachment has advantage but in deciding on this community psychiatric nurses may loose the positive relationship which they may have with a consultant who takes patients from a number of areas. Such working relationships depend largely upon the people involved and they will, in most cases, survive the move away from the idea of a consultant having his 'own' nurse. In the case of geographically based consultants this question should not arise.

Nurses may decide that in order for them to work effectively they must move away from the hospital altogether and become community based. Once again a number of questions will arise. If such a service is organised a decision must be made as to the workings of a referral system and to whom the team is administratively responsible. The team may decide to be attached to health centres or general practitioners moves which will require extensive consultation with the other community disciplines involved. There are obvious benefits to be gained from such a move. The team will be involved more actively in the primary and secondary aspects of psychiatry, but without proper planning the vital contact with the hospital services will be lost. Such a decision, of a hospital or a community base, depends largely on the attitude of the health authority involved. Psychiatric services see themselves either as a central source of psychiatry from which all related services should be directed or they may be of the opinion that the service of psychiatry is a community resource which can be called upon in the event of specialist need. In the former case community psychiatric nurses are more likely to be hospital attached in the latter a community base may be considered.

The traditional psychiatric hospital was built away from the population centres in pleasant countryside. Although in some cases the population has grown out to meet them generally they are still removed from the far ends of their catchment areas and some allowances must be made when organising a community psychiatric nursing service. Catchment areas may be so large that it is necessary to consider mobile day centres which move around the more remote areas and go to meet the community instead of expecting the community to come to the hospital. Such a service could easily have one or two community psychiatric nurses attached to it. Such services are already planned or are in operation Shires (29). Black (30) states the following in response to a survey he undertook in Northumberland:

> The indications from this study are that there is a need to improve patient services in rural Northumberland. It appears that the proposed mobile service will go some way towards these needs.

It is obvious that such a service would not be required in a dense urban setting where a team has a catchment area of a 12 mile radius. Such a service could easily concentrate its resources within a local D.G.H. unit or a centrally positioned day centre and remain accessible to anyone who wished to contact them.

The organisation depends to a great extent on the willingness of divisions of psychiatry to look towards the needs of the community which they serve. The tendency has been to be concentrated in the hospital umbrella and in many cases to be too inward looking. With more constructive thought, a hospital based service can operate with geographical and consultant responsibilities and àt the same time have an outline responsibility towards nominated health centres or G.P. practices within that area.

The essential functioning of a community psychiatric nursing service will be based upon its communications with the patient and his family, the general practitioner, H.V./D.N., consultant psychiatrist, social worker and other interested disciplines. Lines of contact need to be established between the various disciplines and the community psychiatric nursing service. A hierarchical communication channel needs to be organised to ensure that community psychiatric nursing services have access to resources and planning provisions through higher management. A number of alternatives are suitable and two specimen services are shown here with very different but equally effective structures.

Team alpha

This is a hospital based team covering a mixed urban and rural catchment area. The base is within a traditional psychiatric hospital setting. The team take referrals from hospital consultants and will act as an advisory service to the primary health care team. The team does not take permanent cases from the primary health care team without the approval of their consultant who is geographically attached

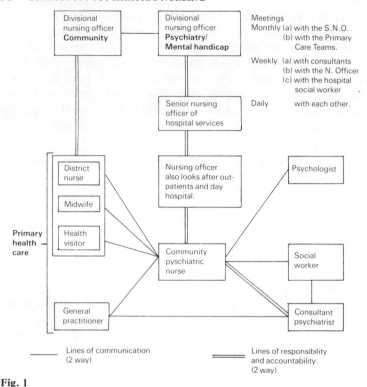

Fig. 1

Discussion of the advantages and disadvantages

Although the community psychiatric nurse is employed and works within the hospital setting the service is still available within a consultative capacity to the primary care team. The consultant psychiatrist has overall control over the decisions about who will be a community psychiatric nursing case and who will not, which tends to weaken the potential of the community psychiatric nursing service. The nursing officer also has responsibility towards the out-patients department and the day hospital which means the community psychiatric nurses feel that they do not get enough of the nursing officer's time. They also feel that the hospital management hierarchy do not have any community experience and therefore do not appreciate the difficulties under which the community psychiatric nurse has to work. The system has the advantage of discussions and policy planning at divisional level as the community psychiatric nurse can feed into both lines of communication. The community psychiatric nurse is seen to be a major link in the communication channels which exist in the psychiatric services. This is an extremely common type of service, relatively easy to run and very little is needed in the way of re-organisation. It is at its most effective when dealing with people who have been through areas such as out-patients, day patients and in-patients. It can provide an effective service as there is easy access to specialist medical services and hospital back-up facilities. There is a close link with the consultant and usually one nurse to each consultant. This closeness can militate against a move towards such things as holding advisory sessions in health centres or being involved in health education as these are not readily seen to be of value. Moves can eventually be made towards these fields but it is usually some time before this happens.

Team beta
This is a community based service with attachment to primary health care teams. The community psychiatric nurses take their referrals from anyone and this covers both hospital and community personnel. The service has a central base and each community psychiatric nurse covers three groups practices/primary care teams. They are geographically organised and take hospital referrals from consultants who are not geographically based. One of the team carries a smaller case load and has nursing officer status.

Discussion of the advantages and disadvantages
The community psychiatric nurses within this service are working

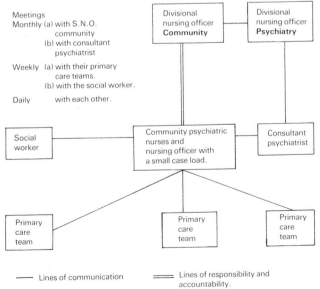

Fig. 2

closely with the primary care teams. When people are discharged from hospital the community psychiatric nurses receive a copy of a discharge letter which is sent to the general practitioner. As this is subject to the usual administrative delays the community psychiatric nurses try to pre-empt this by monthly meetings with the consultant psychiatrist and so they have some idea of who is about to be discharged from hospital. They work much more in the areas of primary and secondary preventive psychiatry and general practitioners refer work which would normally not be adequately covered were there no community psychiatric nursing service available. There is some dissatisfaction within the service and the community psychiatric nurses feel that the community division do not understand enough about psychiatric nursing to run the service effectively and demands are made on the community psychiatric nurses to increase the number of visits made and decrease the time spent on each visit. Although contacts with the hospital are good, the community psychiatric nurses feel 'out on a limb' on occasions. Teams organised along these lines are not quite so common, but a number are operating very efficiently.

The arguments which are postulated here on the 'fors' and 'againsts' of hospital or community base can, under most circumstances be readily sidestepped if community psychiatric nurses are employed by a

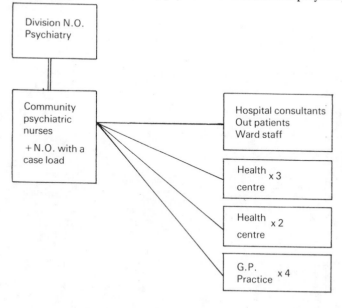

═══ Lines of accountability and responsibility

──── Lines of communication

Fig. 3

psychiatric division, this primarily protects their salary (employment within a community division can mean loss of mental officer status). It would therefore appear to be more sensible to be employed by a psychiatric division. This will of course involve - some hospital referrals. There is no reason why such hospital based community psychiatric nurses should not also have a nominal responsibility towards two or three primary health care teams or G.P. practices. The dichotomy of hospital or community base is then resolved. It is most important to retain contacts with the local hospital services as there is a danger of community psychiatric nurses slipping into the tortures of 'genericism' from which other professional colleagues are now trying to escape!

Community psychiatric nurses have a psychiatric nursing expertise and at the present time a service as outlined here will best serve the community. This is represented diagrammatically in figure 3.

There are bound to be difficulties where divisions of psychiatry do not exist. Under such circumstances sensible placing by nursing management will overcome most difficulties.

All services will develop according to the needs of the population they serve, if provisions are made for the service to be flexible. It may be necessary to have community psychiatric nursing 'out-posts' in distant corners of a large catchment area or to move into the community setting completely. Such things can only be decided by good preparatory discussions and on-going developmental plans.

COMMUNITY PSYCHIATRIC NURSING TEAM MANAGEMENT AND DELIVERY OF SERVICES

The National Health Service is full of the principles of modern management systems which organise and speed up the communications between staff at all levels. What is not quite so well achieved is the effective communication between patient and N.H.S. services. No matter how effective are the communications between professionals and their respective management structures in the N.H.S., a service has failed completely if it is not accessible to, and its objectives understood by, the patient. Nurses often assume that patients are aware of the service that is being offered to them and so do not bother to explain what is available and how to get it. Community psychiatric nurses must not 'assume' that patients know anything about them or the service they offer, and therefore must make provisions which will enable them to be accessible and understood.

Delivery of nursing services

If the delivery of nursing services is to be achieved effectively a number of areas need to be examined.

Initial advertising

A new service needs to make its presence felt. One way of achieving this is to launch a 'promotion exercise'. When the extent and limitations of the service are decided upon and fixed these must be communicated to the other disciplines and community workers. One simple and effective way is to tour services, for example: arrange to see social work area leaders, general practitioners and other primary health care personnel with whom contacts will be essential in future generations. Unless a clear outline is given about the functioning of the community psychiatric nursing service false impressions may be given and the service may be thought of as 'open referral' when it is not intended to be so, and vice versa. If false impressions are given then once communications have broken down future relationships may be adversely affected. Initial impressions are always the most important.

Meeting with other disciplines

These will be essential in the early stages of team development but must be kept in check as they may not be required after the service is off the ground and meetings which serve no useful purpose can be counter-productive.

Explanatory leaflets

If other disciplines and professionals are aware of the existence of the service what about the patient? A leaflet which can outline the aims of the service, also where and how to contact it, are essential to nurse-patient communications. These can be distributed as and when necessary.

Recognised referral system

A structured referral system will make the running of a community psychiatric nursing service easier. It does not matter whether the service is restricted to consultants only, or open to anyone who wished to use it. The referral system must be laid down clearly so that all who are potential users know the system. If the following information is included then it will provide the base for a record system:

> sources of referral;
> name and address of patient, age, sex, diagnosis (if any);
> previous history outline;
> present needs;
> reason for referral.

If such information is available and the community psychiatric nurse then takes up the patient, nursing notes can be added to this base line material. Some skeleton recording system must be set up where the service operates as an open referral service. Recordings must be made of casual involvements as future developments may require some record of what was done and where.

Message leaving service
In a recent survey 10 out of 29 community psychiatric nursing services did not have a telephone number where messages could be left when the community psychiatric nurses were out visiting in the community. This makes nonsense of the idea that a community psychiatric nursing service is available in an 'advisory capacity' and makes the inclusion of 'crisis intervention work' on a job description somewhat suspect. If those seeking advice cannot contact the service at the first try then they may well not bother to do so again. It is essential that a community psychiatric nursing service has a method whereby messages can be left when the community psychiatric nurses are not available. Such a message service should be well publicised and printed onto calling cards which can be left with patients at home.

Hours of working
A flexible approach is needed towards the working hours of the community psychiatric nursing teams. It requires a 'Flexi-hours' system whereby if community psychiatric nurses work late into the evening they can take the hours owing at some other time. This needs an amount of trust between the community psychiatric nurse and their nursing management to get over the possibilities of abuses of this system, however as the working hours of a community psychiatric nurse can be so unpredictable and evening work may be needed to visit working patients, this seems to be the easiest way round the difficulty.

Accessibility
The previous areas could easily be included under accessibility and message leaving and flexible hours are an integral part of being accessible. Other items can also be included. If the community psychiatric nursing service is within a hospital then adequate signs will be needed to guide the patients and other professionals to the community psychiatric nursing site. If a community site is chosen then decisions must be made for central convenience and geographical position.

Transport
Whilst the general feeling is that community psychiatric nurses need their own transportation, methods of remuneration and provision of car loans/cars differ considerably. Shaw(31) found that in the north-west

region 18 per cent of services were provided with cars, 82 per cent were not, 88 per cent of services had access to a cash loan scheme and 12 per cent did not, (this was taken up by 47 per cent of the services).

Car allowances were paid as follows:

    35 per cent claimed flat rates (casual user);

    41 per cent claimed essential rates (regular user);

    18 per cent some claimed flat rate and some claimed essential rate;

    6 per cent some claimed flat rate and some claimed public transport.

In our new re-organised health service the interpretation of what can or cannot be allowed is obviously open to the discretion of administration which is most unsatisfactory. When such discrepancies have been ironed out then services will be able to function much more efficiently.

Team management and relationships

While the preceding area has dealt with wider issues, the team organisation requires consideration. Looking at such items as office practice and relationships can be broken down into component parts.

Relationships

We have already seen that the community psychiatric nursing service can operate from a hospital or community base and some of the relationships involved. There are other relationships which must be cultivated.

Line relationships

This is the hierarchical relationship in which the team will need to be involved to make sure that they are accountable to and accounted for by someone. The question of the role of a nursing officer working within a community psychiatric nursing team is not easily answered. Where they exist, they appear to be of two distinct types:

1. With responsibilities to other areas such as a day hospital and out patients.
2. Where they operate fully within the team and carry a small case load.

The preference would seem to be for type 2 as they are more involved in the specialist needs of community personnel. Where such a separate nursing officer cannot be funded, direct accountability to the senior nursing officer by the community psychiatric nursing team appears to work very well.

Liaisons with other disciplines

If the community psychiatric nursing service is to operate successfully then it must liaise with other professionals in the community. This teamwork is an essential part of the full coverage of the needs of the individual in the community. Certain items lead towards a fuller appreciation of the ingredients of teamwork.

Needs of the individual within the team

Before it is possible to function effectively within a team, each member must have developed certain levels of self-attainment. One important area is that of attitude. Flexibility and awareness of the role of others is essential to the functioning of the team approach. An inflexible team member will produce tension and hostility from others within the team. Confidence in one's own ability is also an essential factor. If challenged or asked for advice, the community psychiatric nurse will need the assuredness and self-confidence to give advice and stand firm on decisions when challenged.

The question of democracy will arise within the team. It is essential to all concerned to know the limitations of team democracy. A distinction which has been refined by Binner (32) as being one of social democracy rather than political democracy. This leads the community psychiatric nurse to the fact that participation in decisions rather than the making of the decisions as a political right will be the order of the day when participating in the team approach. The team needs to appoint a leader in this event, but who this will be is questionable. Some would point automatically to the consultant or the general practitioner as the natural leader. While they may readily take the role on it is not always the wisest choice and some other professional may appropriately be chosen, but without difficulty and feelings of insecurity on the part of other professionals! This decision is very involved in the sensitivity of the team member to the skills and knowledge of other team members.

Needs of the team

The whole team must have an opportunity to comunicate with each other. The isolated meeting of one or two members of the team and unilateral decision-making will produce team fragmentation very quickly. This will necessitate arranging a regular venue which can be as formal as a ward round sessions in the hospital or as informal as a weekly meeting to discuss case difficulties in a community centre.

A periodic review will be essential to see if membership of a particular team serves any useful purpose, if a community psychiatric nurse is, for example, a member of a 'ward round' team which meets once a week, a periodic assessment may show that their presence is superfluous and their time much better served doing other work at that time. Non-participation, because of lack of need, will produce accusations of non-productivity which will lead to dissatisfaction and unrest, therefore a periodic review of the needs of team members will counter this.

A network diagram can indicate the people with whom the community psychiatric nurse will need to create some form of relationship. (See figure 4.)

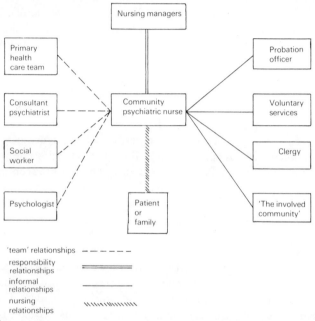

'team' relationships   — — — — — —

responsibility
relationships   ==========

informal
relationships   —————————

nursing
relationships   \\\\\\\\\\\\\\\\\\\\\\\\

Fig. 4

This can only serve to emphasise the great diversity of role expectation which will be placed on the community psychiatric nurse. It therefore serves a a warning to all community psychiatric nurses to sort out their relationships and roles in different situations as they must be aware of the expectations of others upon them.

Collectable statistics
As community psychiatric nursing teams are asked to justify their existences then the need for statistical returns will grow.

Bearing in mind that time is an important factor in the running of a community psychiatric nursing service there are essential statistics which must be collected, as they may prove invaluable in the future planning of a community psychiatric nursing service. These can be listed under simple headings and given to one team member or the responsible nursing officer for tabulation and interpretation.

1. Source of referral. If a service is on offer to all disciplines, this would show which area was not using the service and counter measures could be taken.

2. Name and profession of the associated disciplines. This would show which individuals tend to work closely with the community psychiatric nursing team and which do not.

3. New and re-referrals. Gives some idea of the amount of 'untouched' patients who arrive and an indication to these who use the service repeatedly

4. Those patients who are visited regularly and 'one-offs'. It is important to know what percentage of the community psychiatric nurse's work load is spent on once-only visits, as they are an essential part of the community psychiatric nurse's work. If a caseload is composed of so many regularly visited patients, the provision of once-only visits it severely limits the effectiveness of that service. A survey undertaken in 1973 by the author (33) showed that 26.3 per cent of all visits undertaken by a community psychiatric nursing team were of the once-only category.

To collect statistics which show the effect of community psychiatric nurses on families and the consequent effect of community psychiatric nursing on patients presents a more difficult problem.

Work load assessment
Large case load numbers are not indicative of efficient working methods. Some limitation has to be made on maximum numbers which can be catered for satisfactorily. The thinner the spread of the service the less effective it becomes. The average case load for eighteen services is about 50 patients per nurse in the north-west region, (see Table 4, p. 27). This gives time to visit on a regular basis and allows time for consultation on new cases and 'one-off' visits.

To measure the amount of time needed on each visit is extremely difficult. The variables involved cannot be accounted for as they will fluctuate so greatly. The effects of the present mood of the patient, level of co-operation of patient and family, effectiveness of medication and many other items will all affect the involvement and level of input needed from the community psychiatric nurse. As a result measurement methods used by such bodies as health visitors or district nurses would be totally inappropriate. It would appear that a constant case load of approximately 50 patients who are visited regularly makes a time allowance for these variables and also makes provisions for 'one-off' visits, teaching and administration. If the community psychiatric nurse gets well above this number of patients then a decision must be made to stop taking referrals, even if this is considered to 'endanger' the reputation of the service, competence with limited numbers is better than chaos and inefficiency with large numbers.

Aids to administration

This area can only be talked about where the 'ideal' circumstances exist. This does not occur in all services but they can be borne in mind for a time when more finance is available or made part of a forward budgeting plan.

Secretarial help

This help will clear up two problems with one appointment. Notes will be typed out and kept efficiently and there will be someone there to answer the telephone.

Tape recorders

These provide a means of time-saving between visits consequently allowing more time for the visit itself.

Car radios

These do not constitute a priority rating but serve a very useful purpose in a rural area where to return to base from many miles away only to return out to the same place is costly on time.

Identification

Most services now have a means whereby they can provide each member with a card which will include a photograph of the community psychiatric nurse and a few details about them. Identification is not always asked for, but when needed has to be produced in a convincing format.

REFERENCES

1. Kane, R. A. (1977) *Competency for Collaboration, Current Practice in Family Centred Community Nursing*. Reinhardt, A. M. and Quinn, M. D. (eds) St. Louis: Mosby Company.
   St. Louis: Mosby Company.
2. May, A. R. and Moore, S. (1963) The mental nurse in the community, *The Lancet*, i, 213-214.
3. Greene, J. (1968) The psychiatric nurse in the community, *The International Journal of Nursing Studies*, 5, 175-83.
4. Hunter, P. (1974) Community psychiatric nursing in Great Britain: an historical review, *International Journal of Nursing Studies*, 11, 223-33.
5. Bennet, D. (1964) A community mental health service, *Nursing Times*, December 18th, 1679-80.

6. Harries, C. (1970) Psychiatric nursing and new services for the mentally ill, *Journal of the Nurse Teachers Association*, **1**, Nos. 5 and 6.

7. Altschul, A. T. (1973) A multidisciplinary approach to psychiatric nursing, *Nursing Times*, April 19th.

8. Barker, C. (1977) A community psychiatric nursing service, *Nursing Times*, **73**, No. 28, July 14th.

9. WHO Registered Office for Europe (1971) *Classification and Evaluation of Mental Health Services Activities: Second Interim Report of a Working Group*. Dusseldorf, November 2nd–4th, 1970, Copenhagen.

10. WHO (1975) *Working Group on the Role of Nursing in Psychiatric and Mental Health Care*. Saarbrucken, March, 1975. ICP/MNH 139(S).

11. D.H.S.S. (1975) *Better Services for the Mentally Ill*. Cmmnd. No. 6233.

12. Shore, A. (1977) Shore, A. An appraisal of the existing C.P.N. services in the N.W. region. *Community Psychiatric Nursing Research Monograph*, No. 19, Manchester Polytechnic.

13. Hicks, D. (1976) *Primary Health Care*. London: H.M.S.O.

14. Shepherd, M., Cooper, B., Brown, A. C., and Kalton, G. (1966) *Psychiatric Illness in General Practice*. London: Oxford University Press.

15. Watts, C. A. H. (1962) *Studies on Medical and Population Subjects*, No. 14. London: H.M.S.O.

16. Driver, E. (1976) Assessment of the demand for a C.P.N. service in Chester, Manchester Polytechnic *Community Psychiatric Nursing Research Monograph* No. 1.

17. Leopoldt, H. (1975) Hospital based community psychiatric nursing psychogeriatic care, *Nursing Mirror*, December, 18th.

18. H.M.S.O. (1970) *Psychiatric Case Registers*, D.H.S.S. Statistical Report. Series. No. 8.

19. H.M.S.O. (1971) *The Nottingham Psychiatric Case Register Findings 1962–1969*. Statistical Report Series, No. 13.

20. Hull, D. J., Robertson, N. C., Olley, P. C. and Millar, W. M. (1973) The north-east Scottish psychiatric case register—the second phase, *Journal of Chronic Disorders*, **26**, 375.

21. Sainsbury, P. (1976) The problems of evaluation a community psychiatric service, *Community Development Journal*, **11**, No. 3.

22. Kessel, N. (1968) The whirligig of time: a cautionary tale. In *Community Mental Health*. Williams, R. H. and Ozarin, L. O. (eds). pp. 500–507. Jersey Press.

23. Warren, J. (1971). Long acting Phenothrazine injections given by psychiatric nurses in the community, *Nursing Times*, September. pp. 141–43.

24. White, D. M. D. (1973) Organising psychogeriatric care in the community. *Nursing Times*, January 18, 97–98.

25. Willey, R. (1969) Nursing after-care in society. *Nursing Times*, **65**, 1629.

26. Henderson, J. G. (1973) The role of the psychiatric nurse in domicilliary treatment service, *Nursing Times*, **69**, 1334–1378.

27. Leopoldt, H. (1973) Psychiatric community nursing, *Social Services Journal*, **83**, 489–90.

28. Hacker, P., Leopoldt, H., and Robinson, J. R. (1976) Attaching C.P.N.s to general practice, *Journal of R.C.G.P.*, **36**, 666–71.

29. Shires, J. (1977) A travelling day hospital—an experiment in rural community care, *Social Work Today*, **8**, No. 24. March 23rd.

30. Black, J. (1977) Feasibility of introducing a mobile psychiatric service in rural Northumberland, *Manchester Polytechnic Community Psychiatric Nursing Monograph*, No. 13.

31. (Cf. 12 supra)

32. Binner, P. (1967) The team and the concept of democracy, *Journal of the Fort Logan Mental Health Centre*, **4**, 115–24.

33. Butterworth, C. A. (1973) The case for a community psychiatric team, *Manchester Polytechnic Psychiatric Nursing Monograph*, No. 51.

4

The emergence and development of the community mental handicap nursing team

The services for the mentally handicapped have been traditionally associated with those of psychiatry and to confuse one with the other is still not uncommon, even amongst professional people involved in care. It is, however, a link which is largely historical; the uneasy marriage vacillates between break-up and reconciliation with interested parties attempting to push the liaison in the direction their own philosophy of care demands. Mental handicap is not a clinical entity or a diagnostic category. The title covers a wide range of behaviours including slow development or slow learning, social incompetence, difficulty with simple arithmetic or complex movements—but is questionably psychiatric or medical. The care of the mentally handicapped and the development of the community services has reflected this difficulty of categorisation with the educational, social and medical services being involved.

THE WHEEL TURNS FULL CIRCLE

The concept of mental handicap is largely culturally and socially determined. Some of the handicaps now prevalent would not have survived in earlier times, such is medical progress, whilst others would have been unnoticed in a less sophisticated age. It is interesting however, that one of the main points of interest for community care, the pre-school child and his early educational stimulation, is not fundamentally different from the scheme devised to socialise and educate 'Victor' the 'wild boy of Aveyron' by Dr. Itard in 1801, which led to the philosophy that 'The Idiot may be Educated'. Victor was trained through the senses, not altogether unsuccessfully to live in a domestic environment. The other major area of interest, the restoration to the community people previously segregated from it, results from a later philosophy that dictated that only care for life could efficiently treat feebleness of the mind.

Early concepts of community care

It was perhaps unfortunate that the Colonies set-up to segregate the mentally deficient became hospitals in 1948 which has left us with the legacy of medical domination and the medical model of care.

The Mental Health Act of 1959 encouraged the movement towards community care for the mentally subnormal (in the terminology of the act) consisting of junior training centres where self-help skills, sense-training, communication and motor skills were intended to be developed. The senior training centre catered for the adult. Here the emphasis was on a manual-work orientated approach, with a predominance of repetitive assembly-type tasks being undertaken. Both centres were the responsibility of the Health Department. The act was however a permissive one, and the opportunities afforded were taken up with differing degrees of enthusiasm by the local authorities. Some made use of existing training facilities in old mansions and other buildings in various states of repair; others, like the west riding of Yorkshire built many new centres with junior and senior centres usually on the same site. This has subsequently caused problems with the redistribution of responsibility and the expansion of the services offered. The other mainstay of the community services as they were envisaged at the time was the hostel. The Wood Committee, 1929 had already mooted the half-way-house principle but it was not much in evidence. (Sheffield had a hostel for women in 1942.) The hostel programme was again undertaken with varying degrees of enthusiasm. However, many were satellite hospitals in the community but not integrated, and still retained all the hallmarks of institutional care. The only person giving a personal service was the duly authorised officer who became the mental health officer of the 1959 Mental Health Act. This service was mainly one of making contact, the officer being largely seen as a figure of authority.

Cracks in the wall

From 1948 the responsibility for the mentally handicapped lay with the health authorities. In the late 1960s, pressure was mounting to expunge Section 57 of the 1944 Education Act and to integrate the mentally handicapped into the mainstream of education. The Education (Handicapped Children) Act of 1970 came into effect on April 1st, 1971. The junior training centre became the special school and responsibility was transferred to the educational authorities. Overall responsibility for the senior training centres was transferred to the Social Services Department under the Social Services Act, 1971. The 1972 white paper 'Better services for the mentally handicapped'(1) further encouraged the development of community services endorsing the principle of 'normalisation' and the 'right of every mentally handicapped person to live among us'. Strangely, the British Association of Social Workers, in its policy statement 'Better services for the mentally handicapped' 'regrets that the white paper does not come down firmly in favour of small units attached to District General Hospitals'. This policy statement of B.A.S.W. reflects the attitude of many a social worker that mental handicap is vaguely medical.

Mental handicap and the nurses role

Mental handicap, although historically linked with psychiatry, has a different history. The development of the service reflects the indecisiveness of whom should be primarily responsible. The nurses in the field of mental handicap have been expressing concern about their future when the emphasis is on community care and have taken a long time to appreciate that, because the size of the hospital in terms of beds has been diminishing, the mentally handicapped do not just disappear. The nurses have been aware that the number of mentally handicapped people living outside of hospitals exceeds those living within, yet have only lately taken an interest in whether these people need the help of the only group of professional people specifically trained to care for the handicapped. Should the specialist mental handicap nurse be the person to be working in the community at all? Does the nurse of the mentally handicapped have a future? The long term answer may be 'no', but in the short term a person adequately prepared to support families in the areas they need—day to day management and self help—skilled training is urgently required.

ORIGINS OF THE PRESENT SERVICE

Links between the hospital and the community have in the past been limited and tenuous, often relying on a single social worker or the informal links retained by the staff of hospitals and hostels as their patients were discharged, keeping a friendly or fatherly eye on their progress. In a survey carried out in 1966, the Royal Medical Psychological Association found eight hospitals for the mentally handicapped employed a total of eight nurses full time and twenty-five part time, mainly for follow-up and social work. The formal development of a community service is, however, of recent origin. Some hospitals have highly developed services; many are in the process of expanding services to make them more comprehensive but as yet there is no firm agreement on role, elements of care carried out willingly in one service being derided in another as not being nurses' work.

In a survey reported in 1974(2) Strong and Sandland found the following types of service in operation:

1. Finding employment and accommodation.
2. Social education.
3. Pre-admission visits.
4. Home visiting of in-patients relatives.
5. Out-patient clinics.
6. Community liaison officer.

The community nursing services at present vary widely. Some are very institutionally-orientated with a concentration on pre-admission, post-discharge visits, follow up from out-patients clinics, depot injections, making regular contact visits to iron out problems or offering short term care. 'Most hospitals have developed a short term care system affording valuable relief to families, but in many cases this is the limit of their contribution to the care of the mentally handicapped living in the community' (Baker(3)). This report goes on to say 'The importance of an out-patient service for family support and counselling, out-patient treatment, and follow-up of rehabilitated patients cannot be over-stressed and should be accorded an equal priority to the improvement of in-patient facilities'.

Some area health authorities would deem the community nurse for the mentally handicapped is only of any relevance for the over sixteen year old, whereas others see the support of families as being of prime importance. Support in this instance meaning advice on day to day management and care, and intensive home teaching.

> A particular problem, largely overlooked at present, is to provide practical advice for parents and in particular mothers of young mentally handicapped children about problems of behaviour and development. I am not referring to counselling here, the importance of which is widely recognised, but to practical advice on the management of the handicapped children to help families to cope with the unusual and difficult problems of children who are *different* from others. Parents can't get advice from relatives, friends and other mothers about such children, since their experience will be no greater than their own. They need specialist help.
>
> J. Tizard(4)

Is it a nursing service?
As with the community psychiatric nurse (for the mentally ill) there is a degree of overlap between professionals working in the field. Some would argue that 'the mentally deficient person whether he is an infant, child, adolescent or an adult is firstly a human being and secondarily mentally deficient. Though he may require specialised services his basic needs are similar to those of other people in our society.' G. Tarjan, and T. L. Pilkington(10, 11) states 'The mentally handicapped do not form a homogeneous clinical group, and the

educational, social, and medical needs of most of them should be met as an extension of the services provided for the ordinary population'.

EARLY EDUCATION SCHEMES

In this context the educational home visiting of the educational priority area research project in the west riding of Yorkshire in 1970 was probably the first scheme intended for parents to promote the development of their children. 'The early visitors were usually trained teachers operating from a nursery or infant school. Increasingly other professionals—nursery nurses, playgroup leaders, social workers— and volunteers have been engaged in visiting schemes.' This is the view of the National Children's Bureau(5).

In 1971, the Hester Adrian Research Centre (Manchester University) organised 'workshops' for parents of mentally handicapped children, 'The courses are primarily aimed at helping the parent help the child. We believe that the greatest need of many parents is to feel that they are doing something to help their own child and are not totally reliant upon professionals.' Cunningham and Jeffree(6).

The workshops were intended for parents of children, rather than adolescents or adults, and, significantly, no representative of social class 4 or 5—where the degree of under stimulation and corresponding under achieving are likely to be greater—attended. The Hester Adrian Centre now has one focus amongst many on the role of the health visitor in early intervention with Down's syndrome babies (see Community outlook, *Nursing Times* June 8th, 1978).

Specialised programmes for the equivalent of the health visitor in America, the public health nurse, have already been developed for P.H.N.s in Salt Lake City, Utah. 'It is my hypothesis that the public health nurse who acquires additional education and skill is the most logical person to provide early home-centred stimulation for infants.' A. B. Godfrey(7).

Athleen Godfrey then set up a training scheme for public health nurses in early stimulation programmes.

In Arizona, F.I.N.D. (First Identification of Neonatal Disabilities) is a programme to provide a counsellor available to physicians and other agencies when the condition of mental retardation is diagnosed. It is a service intended to be available to the family from the day of birth.

F.I.N.D. will:

1. Offer weekly staff visits in your home.
2. Offer a fundamental learning programme from 9.00 a.m. to 2.30 p.m. daily.

3. Give advice and information about resources available to the mentally retarded.
4. Do everything possible from birth to see that the child in question receives whatever services are necessary to help the individual develop to his potential.
5. Give the mother and family whatever help is necessary in planning for the development of the new child.
6. Make referrals to appropriate agencies.

These programmes, as with the admirable work of Janet Carr in London, Cliff Cunningham in Manchester and the Developmentally Young project of the Hester Adrian Centre are concerned with very young children with emphasis on their development delay. These may be seen as very necessary preventative measures. How significantly the Sheffield Development Project states 'The study team have not counted the question of prevention as part of their remit ...'. The study did acknowledge the need for early detection and educational stimulation but relying rather too heavily on nursery classes and day nurseries and a comprehensive assessment by a multidisciplinary team. Whilst being essential services thère remains the less severely handicapped, the child who behaves 'differently' and the child who becomes adolescent and adult. Who now advises? It is here the community nurse with a special interest in mental handicap is most useful. (The unfortunate connotation in the minds of parents of the word 'nurse' does present somewhat of a problem as 'nursing' is not what the parents feel they require. A suitable alternative title has not been forthcoming.) It is in the area of practical help on the management of severely handicapped people that the nurse has a role. In the words of Athleen Godfrey 'an integration of occupational and physical therapy techniques, behaviour shaping and developmental concepts, and a dash of imagination'. Until some of the recommendations of the Court Committee (Fit for the Future) are implemented this combination of skills belongs to the appropriately trained nurse of the mentally handicapped. The health visitor is not currently prepared to accept the role.

TYPES OF SERVICE

The community service must, of necessity, undertake the preventive aspects of care associated with the developmentally young, it must give practical help and advice to parents to enable them to care for their children at home whilst offering periodic short term care facilities to give a break, relieve a crisis or allow parents to attend a social function. The advice may need to be on such areas as nutrition, health care, toy selection and the use of toy libraries as well as modification of unacceptable behaviour.

The community nursing service for the mentally handicapped being of recent origin, although having similar aims and principles do differ, and, what is more, fail to agree on the role of the nurse within the community. Two particular areas of disagreement are job finding and 'baby-sitting'. The former is thought by many to be a function of the social worker although it forms a major component of some services, and the latter regarded by some people as a waste of nursing skills, whereas for other areas this comprises a widely appreciated major function. The notion that nurses should roll up their sleeves and give practical help causes concern in some nurses who see their primary role as counselling. Some would prefer to give parental advice on coping rather than to become actively involved. There are enough curb-side-foremen already—let's have people in the service who are prepared to give the help required by the mentally handicapped and their families.

Families will develop a strategy of care, some strategies may not, however, be in the best interests of the mentally handicapped person or the family. The tendency to treat as a child, often in the past encouraged by professionals, will require a change of attitude through education, and skilful counselling and support through the period of insecurity that may ensue. The mentally handicapped adolescent will experience similar problems to the normal adolescent. The intellectual deficit and slow learning of socially relevant ways of behaving may present additional difficulties and the physical, and emotional changes and sexual interest that develops should not be circumvented by the dubious tactic of encouraging perpetual dependence. Young adults commonly move away from home; the mentally handicapped adult should have the right to live away from home, if he or she wishes to do so. Suitable accommodation ought therefore to be provided and habilitation programmes be implemented to encourage the development of independent living to the extent that this is possible. These programmes and the monitoring of progress are an important function of the community nurse.

From hospital to community

Consideration needs also to be given to the people in hospitals for the mentally handicapped who do not require the specialist services a hospital can offer and could adequately live in accommodation graded in terms of the degree of supervision afforded. Social training programmes have been part of the hospital scene for some time. Rehabilitated patients should have had the benefit of a well devised rehabilitation programme but the community nurse ought to be aware that this will not always be the case.

Once placed in a community, the people discharged from hospital will require regular, yet hopefully diminishing, contact with someone from the place in which which they have spent much of their lives. This would smooth the transition to integrated living as part of a community—rather than apart from society—a situation with which they would be more familiar. Close liaison needs to be maintained between the rehabilitation wards, the hostels and half-way houses, as well as the schools, occupational and training centres, all of whom organise social training programmes.

The placing of former inmates of mental handicap institutions in the community does not find universal favour. 'If patients are going to be happier in the community then integrate them into the community, but the majority of patients are far happier in hospital, living in the environment they know.' Mr Crawford(8) is not alone in making such assumptions, I know not on what evidence. Anecdotal evidence of people who have spent many years in typically custodial care has shown they adjust far more quickly to living in the community than one would hope or expect. It rather depends on the manner of the transfer.

In his article 'Community as dustbin', Michael Clarke(9) begins:

> The community is increasingly being used as a healing agency for all social ills. Criminals, juvenile delinquents, addicts, the old, the mentally disordered, the handicapped—all are supposed to benefit from a return to the community.

Later he goes on to state:

> Patients who improve are turned out of the hospital usually with no friends, few relations in contact, and little prospect of employment, to remain in a community they cannot find until they become sufficiently troublesome to those who are in contact with them to be returned to hospital.

Such a situation would not occur if patients are adequately prepared for living and there is a systematic programme of continuing support.

It is important that people previously overprotected within an institutional setting are cushioned for a while from the hazards of living within a society for which they cannot be adequately prepared. One has no wish to transfer the overprotective nature of the institution to the community, yet the rehabilitated patient will encounter stress heretofore unfamiliar and may react in ways somewhat less than desirable. Social life, in fact life in total, has been supplied by the hospital. The tendency to withdraw from contact with others when placed in a situation where friendship has to be gained and pleasure sought rather than being gratuitously supplied is strong. The community nurse is in the best position to gauge the effects of community living on the mentally handicapped. It is no restoration of human dignity to be subject to unwarranted stress in the name of community care. It is not a successful rehabilitation if the mentally handicapped person is apparently coping rather than coping in reality.

TEAM SIZE AND ORGANISATION

The case-load that can be carried by the community nurse will vary with the type of service provided and the locality in which it is situated, urban or rural. The case-loads vary from over 100 to under 30. A case.load of 50 results in a 'contact service': 'Hello, how are you? I haven't time for tea, see you next week', which is abusing the title 'community care'. The nurse in the community must demonstrate her special skills, giving practical and, if necessary, intensive assistance to those who require it, which means keeping case-loads small.

A regular review of case-loads will be required. Long term infrequent maintenance visiting, a function crisis-orientated social workers do less well, is a necessary part of the nurses role. She should also monitor behavioural and social functioning, including the effectiveness of drugs or side effects, and ensure that the people rehabilitated from institutions, who may not be aware of such things as unemployment benefit, know what to do about insurance claims or exaggerated bills, and are not unduly stressed. Early recognition of a potential breakdown would avoid unnecessary readmissions. A periodic re-evaluation of the 'Nursing' input is required to avoid the growth of excessive case-loads and to reduce the problem of client dependency. There must come a time however, when if social competence is taken as the major criterion for mental retardation, the person should not be so regarded when they become socially competent.

The teams at present in operation vary from a single charge nurse to a team of nine led by a senior nursing officer. A team of three or four of which one may be a nursing officer seems the most common. The presence of the nursing officer should reduce the administrative load of the individual charge nurses, gives access to the nursing administration to a person with working knowledge of the service, encourages staff development and training, and gives the beginnings of a career structure. It is important that the nursing officer carries a case-load, reduced to take account of his managerial and training responsibilities.

Some areas, whilst awaiting further developments following the imminent publication of the Peggy Jay Report on the future pattern of staff training for the care of the mentally handicapped, are putting out tentative feelers towards forming a community team as set out in pamphlet no. 2 from the National Development Group. This pamphlet suggests the setting up of community mental handicap teams consisting of a core team of a nurse and a social worker (or other specialist) for a locality, three such teams being supported by professional staff, (psychologist, mental handicap consultants, speech and physiotherapists) hospital and residential services. The national development group believe that each team should be able to cater for a population of between 60 000–100 000 which would result in the average N.H.S. District of 200 000–250 000 people would need two or three core teams and supporting services.

The setting up of such teams would be a useful development from the present somewhat fragmented situation. A further development would be the organisation of a district handicap team consisting of consultant community paediatrician, nursing officer for handicapped children, specialist social worker, psychologist and teacher as outlined in the Court Report ('Fit for the future'). 'The Team would provide a special diagnostic assessment and treatment service for children with all kinds of handicap including the severely retarded. Specialist services for these children should in the Committee's view no longer be so sharply differentiated from those of more intelligent children.'

Such teams may well be some time in the future. Meantime, the development of a team of nurses with a degree of specialism, in the care of the elderly mentally handicapped, the adolescent, children or behaviour disorders and their management, would provide the team with improved advice, lead to an improved service to the client, encourage further progress and prepare a sound base on which to build the multidisciplinary community teams.

The future of nursing education in the field of mental handicap is at present uncertain. To anticipate the Peggy Jay Report requires a degree of crystal gazing. The education of the professionals should result in a move away from the medically orientated model of care previously prevalent, a move away from the link so often made with general psychiatry and towards multidisciplinary courses at basic and post-basic level. Large parts of the present service administered by the Health Service may become the responsibility of other departments as many people who are mentally handicapped presently living in hospital do not need to be there for reasons of health or require the specialist services only available in hospital. The generally acknowledged gap in the present service is the provision of experienced skilled help to the families and the handicapped person at home. This gap urgently needs to be closed and the future education should reflect this need.

Operational setting of the community nursing team

The setting for the community nursing team will reflect the philosophy underpinning the service to be provided and the locality in which the service will operate. Placing the team within the hospital has a number of attractions, it will be close to the specialised resources that reside in hospitals—physiotherapists, doctors, psychologists, medical technology and sophisticated assessment procedures, as well as being able to derive support from the nursing service. The hospital based team would be aware of the general and special functions and facilities of the hospital, and have some knowledge about the patients whose discharge is imminent and be able to follow up more easily patients they themselves had a hand in admitting. Access to beds is an area generating some discussion. Some psychiatrists have a pre-occupation with maintaining power over admissions and whilst it is not always difficult to obtain permission to admit, it would be preferable if the example of the more enlightened areas where nurses, and in some cases psychologists, have access to beds without recourse to medical authority was followed. The access issue may be better for the hospital based team although experience would indicate that it depends on the orientation and attitude of the consultant rather than on where the team is based.

The hospital based team may be disadvantaged by the institutional conservative attitudes that accompany large hospitals. This situation is made worse where the team has responsibilities within the parent hospital for habilitation or pre-discharge units. The dual responsibility has a tendency to weight the priorities towards discharge rather than giving a service which prevents admission by giving parents and families adequate support. Within an unenlightened hospital, time is devoted to defending the service against critics often in influential positions. This time could be more profitably spent thinking creatively about service development.

Placing the team at a location outside the large hospitals poses problems and benefits. Where the team is to be housed will depend on the locality, its facilities and administrative structure. A team based on a 'community centre' may be more remote from the hospital and specialist services, but will be closer to those for whom it exists, its *raison d'etre*. Being distanced from supportive services the nurse will be in a stronger position to develop professional skills at the same time, being close to the community served, will be in a better position to be aware of local needs. Problems may arise through being out of touch with mainstream mental handicap and keeping up to date with trends in mental handicap or developments of a capital or administrative nature but are not insurmountable. Nurses based within the community are more likely to be accepted for their specialist nursing skills which will then be utilised, than their proximity to hospital on the erroneous assumption that admission will be all the easier.

Re-organisation of the health and local authorities, subsequent re-thinks on the original arrangements and the sectorisation of authority areas makes the choice of site difficult. The community nurse could be linked to a number of primary health care teams covering a geographical area, operating from a day centre, hostel or other centre; it is unfortunate that the sectors of the social services are not usually co-terminous. The present preference for a district based service results in only one district in an area receiving a service or where two district-based services exist, the organisational structure and philosophy are so different as to cause confusion within the social services and the families for whom the service is intended. It is a fear that the district-based services will be so busy liaising with each other and the social workers whose different geographical areas overlap, that the service to families suffers as a result. There is a danger that a communications network is set up operating at a number of different levels yet leaving holes through which the client falls unsupported. This problem will be exaggerated when a patient is discharged from hospital in which he has lived for a number of years yet chooses to live in a part of a town for whom another district has responsibility. Policy may and does vary on the type of service provided and the balance to be maintained between family support follow up visits or the gathering of information.

An area health authority-based service co-terminous as it is with the local authority boundaries would seem the most appropriate. It is an historical accident that many hospitals are badly placed in relation to their catchment area, in some rural areas it may be necessary for the community team to be mobile. It is unfortunate that administrators think in terms of buildings rather than services. A mobile community service could have a set pattern of visiting, supporting and complementing existing services in the community plus an office where messages may be taken for requests for assistance that cannot be met by the peripatetic team or where a personal call would be more appropriate.

Referrals
These too are affected by the philosophy of the service. Some nurses (for reasons beyond comprehension) seem to delight in the 'hand-

maiden-to-doctor' role, circulating with due reverence like acolytes. This results in a consultant dominated service with consultant referral. The more enlightened services have adopted an open referral system whereby people (including professionals) requiring assistance can contact the nurse as a professional in her own right. A professional attitude brings professional responsibilities and this must be reflected in the acceptance of such cases as can be competently handled with the available resources, avoiding the unnecessary building up of case-loads.

The Community Nursing Service for the mentally handicapped, although having similarities, has a different history and, hopefully, a different future to the role of the community psychiatric nurse, yet they share the experience, excitement and problems of growing as a profession.

REFERENCES

1. B.A.S.W. (1974) Better Services for the Mentally Handicapped. B.A.S.W.'s Policy.
2. Strong, P. G. and Sandland, E. T. (1974) Subnormality nursing in the community, *Nursing Times*, March 7th.
3. Baker, A. A. (1972) Annual Report of the Hospital Advisory Service.
4. Tizard, J. (1972) *Mental Handicap 1947-1972*. Address given to the National Society for Mentally Handicapped Children Convention and Annual Conference, April 29th, 1972.
5. National Childrens Bureau Information Service. Highlight No. 29 (1977).
6. Cunningham, C. C. and Jeffree, D. M. (1975) The organisation and structure of workshops for parents of mentally handicapped children, *Bulletin of British Psychology*, **28**, 405-11.
7. Godfrey, A. B. (1975) Sensory-motor stimulation for slow-to-develop children, *American Journal of Nursing*, **75**, No. 1, January.
8. Crawford, D (1972) Community care and the mentally handicapped, *Nursing Times*, June 8th.
9. Clarke, M. (1976) Community as dustbin, *New Society*, July 29th.

5

Strategies for care in community psychiatric nursing

COMMUNITY PSYCHIATRIC NURSING

Community nursing of the mentally disordered presents a new and challenging approach for those working within the community. It places demands on the nurse to demonstrate skills which have hitherto been under-utilised in the more formal, traditional setting of institutional care. The move into the community requires a shift in the knowledge base to prepare the nurse to work with people in their own home without the support and security of the hospital with its customary roles, rituals and routines. Community nursing will require a considerable amount of introspection and change especially in the areas of nurse–patient relationships, roles and attitudes.

The most startling yet unobvious change is from that of a group to an individualistic approach. The mere fact of being in the patient's home where he is on his own, where he can more easily be appreciated as a person, as an individual and different to everyone else, is so obvious that it can easily be missed; and yet it is one of the fundamental changes which is experienced by those nurses moving from hospital to community work. In the hospital setting the nurse/patient role is clearly defined and the expectations of each upon the other is well mapped out. In the community these expectations alter, where nurses were once the masters of the situation other factors are at play. You are a visitor in someone's house and as such, immediately disadvantaged compared with the ward sister/charge nurse position in the hospital situation.

New strategies for care are required, from the medical concepts of curative care to the more all-embracing concepts of preventative care, from training the patient to teaching the family, from an inward-looking institutional centralising of resources to using the variable scattered community resources and from an institutional to a patient-orientated pattern of care, based more closely on the perceived needs of the client. The areas of social psychiatry, psychotherapy and behaviour therapy are discussed elsewhere in the book. This section however, will endeavour to look at some of the current thinking in both nursing and the care of the mentally disordered generally. It is not intended to dictate which areas or strategies should be adopted, rather to give an insight into areas which the community psychiatric nurse may wish to use or study in more detail.

STRATEGIES

THE COMMUNITY PSYCHIATRIC NURSE AND THE NURSING PROCESS

There is a considerable amount of literature (predominantly American) on the nursing process. It has been variously described as:

> A dynamic, on-going interpersonal process in which nurse and patient are viewed as a system with each affecting the behaviour of the other and both being affected by factors within the situation. (1)
> A process by which a nurse acts while responsible for the care of patients (2)

Perhaps one of the most useful is that of Mayers:

> A rational and systematic process with intellectual, behavioural and technical elements based on theories from behavioural and physical sciences. (3)

The nursing process is not confined to any one area of specialist nursing such as surgery or psychiatry, but serves as a useful framework to examine nursing carried out in a variety of settings. It has, however, something special to offer community psychiatric nurses.

One of the major objectives of the nursing process is to work towards individualised patient care. In an institutional setting this can pose difficulties as the nursing process places emphasis on one to one nurse–patient relationship and all the demands on staffing levels that this would present. The community psychiatric nurse is in an enviable position. The very nature of their work demands that patients are being seen on an individualised basis and we need not concern ourselves with this area, other than to stress the important point that nurses can sometimes be in danger of approaching patients as 'Schizophrenics' or 'Mongols' and the nursing process applied to community psychiatric nursing demands that even this approach be stopped. Patients need to be approached as individuals who have needs which the nurse can either supply or help the patients to supply for themselves. This may require a considerable amount of attitude change on the part of the nurse, as this exercise demands an objective rather than a subjective approach. Assuming then, that the individualised approach is satisfied it is possible to look in more detail at the nursing process.

The nursing process can be divided into five basic stages. These can then be broken down further into more detailed elements:

Stage one

Information gathering
In the establishment of a working relationship with a patient the community psychiatric nurse has to collect, sort and collate important information needed for achieving initial assessment and future evaluation of progress. Three important elements in this area are:

1. Investigation. When a patient is referred to the community psychiatric nurse there are sources of investigation where the community psychiatric nurse can glean useful information—i.e. case notes, G.P.'s records, ward kardex, social work reports, this will not only provide essential case and background information, but also provides contact with other caring agencies who may be involved.

2. Interviewing. The initial interview is a vitally important time for both the community psychiatric nurse and the patient in establishing a working relationship. The basic material exchanged will affect the future development of such things as mutual trust and communication. It is not the purpose of this chapter to examine in detail the art of interviewing, but it is useful to remember such points as having the right setting for the interview, turning up punctually for the interview, accurate recording of the information received, and the dynamics of the interviewer/interviewee relationship.

3. Observation. It should be obvious to the psychiatric nurse that one of the skills which they should have developed continually after basic training and post basic experience is in the area of observation. The skilled observer is looking at the 'clues' and 'cues' given by patients in both their verbal and non-verbal behaviour.

Throughout our information gathering stage the community psychiatric nurse using the three elements previously outlined should have gained information on:

a. Personal characteristics
Age, sex, marital status, occupation, ethnic or cultural origins, physical difficulties or disabilities.

b. Levels of functioning
Perceptions of reality, self-image, personal integrity, ego functioning, psychosocial development, social-cultural supplies, family involvement etc.

c. Presenting difficulties with themselves
What do they think is wrong? What do others think is wrong with them? Why did they seek help? How did the caring agencies become involved?

Stage Two

Assessment of needs
The community psychiatric nurse should have a picture of the patient through which it is possible to assess strengths and weaknesses. As with a physical disability it is possible to build onto existing strengths to help to minimise deficiencies or weaknesses in other areas.   With the information received in the three identified areas of personal characteristics, levels of functioning and presenting difficulties to the community psychiatric nurse, should be able to analyse the needs of that particular patient, not as an 'illness' but as a person with 'needs'. These may be areas in which the nurse may have to be the 'surrogate self' or take over part of that person's functioning until they can satisfactorily perform it themselves and this is where a 'nursing diagnosis' would be made. Examples of this are given in the two case studies.

Stage Three

Formulation of a plan of care
The production of a nursing care plan is very much the choice of the individual community psychiatric nurse. It will vary with every patient the community psychiatric nurse deals with, but there are stages through which all care plans must go.

1. Priority listing. The community psychiatric nurse has to decide on a priority rating for the items listed under their assessment of that patient's needs, i.e. is resocialisation more important than establishing a regular balanced diet?

2. Choice of nursing care. The community psychiatric nurse will examine the priorities which have been set and decide on the approach needed; i.e. physical care, supportive psychotherapy, health education—whichever is the most appropriate method for the task.

3. Organisation. This will identify the timing of the nursing care provided and will be needed at any particular time.

Goal setting will be a major factor in this area, i.e. 'in five weeks an attempt will have been made to alter phobic behaviour which is characterised by an inability to go into local shops'. A review date can be set at the time to monitor the progress which has or has not been made.

Stage Four

Implementation of a care plan
Decisions have been made by the community psychiatric nurse about the needs of a particular patient and how the nursing care will be

applied to these needs in an effort to meet them when the care plan is implemented the community psychiatric nurse is going to be involved in using a variety of skills—technical and basic skills, interaction skills and observation skills.

It is not necessary to follow the plan rigidly. The nurse will be using the cognitive functions of perception and judgement and circumstances may demand the rejection of a particular care plan or its modification to suit change in behaviour or circumstances.

Stage Five

Evaluation
There is a need for evaluation in any process undertaken by the community psychiatric nurse. The nurse will need to know what changes in the patient's status have taken place and whether these were for the better or for the worse. If changes have been made which have adversely affected the patient then these will show up on evaluation and if present require some form of change in the plan. It may be that the goal setting was aimed too high and in an effort to achieve, the patient may have been overstressed, thus making progress impossible. This would require a modification in (1) time span allowed for levels of achievement or (2) reduction into more elemental stages of the behaviour change or developmental level being attempted.

Success also needs to be measured. When a relationship is established and the nurse and the patient meet on a regular basis it is not always easy to remember the progress which has been made towards satisfying the patients needs. Success tends to breed more success and can be a useful spur to both the nurse and the patient.

One other item of importance in this area is that of the possibility of terminating a relationship. If success has been nil, or the objectives of the care plan have been fully met, then the relationship may need to be terminated. Nurses have often not been taught the art of terminating a relationship and when or why to do it. Evaluation provides a method of deciding on whether or not continuing the relationship is of value to the patient.

The nursing process can provide a system through which the community psychiatric nurses can organise their nursing care. It provides a planned system with objective goals and consciously uses the cognitive skills which are used by the nurse when provided with factual observed data.

The two following case studies have been subjected to the nursing process and provide examples of working through problems which the community psychiatric nurse may possibly come across.

Case study A

A written request was received from a consultant psychiatrist by the community psychiatric nurse to 'visit' the following patient after discharge and to 'support and maintain effective medication in the community'.

Diary of events prior to patient's discharge and after referral to the community psychiatric nurse

1. January 12th   Admitted to hospital
2. February 18th   Referred to community psychiatric nurse (one week prior to discharge)
3. February 19th   Patient interviewed by community psychiatric nurse on the ward
4. February 21st   Husband interviewed at home
5. February 22nd   Care plan formulated
                   G.P. informed by community psychiatric nurse of imminent discharge
6. February 25th   Discharged home, care of community psychiatric nurse
7. February 25th   Visited by community psychiatric nurse and care plan implemented
8.   Visited as per care plan
9. March 24th   Care plan evaluated and adjusted.

Information from case notes

Psychiatric consultation was required after an obvious deterioration in the mental stability of Mrs X. She was becoming withdrawn and agitated, showing distinct episodes of paranoia against her immediate neighbours. She accused them of interfering with her property and talking about her amongst themselves. A diagnosis of late paraphrenia with a possible concomitant dementing process was made.

Nursing kardex information

The ward nursing kardex stated that Mrs X was visited regularly by her husband but no one else. She was encouraged to join in the ward social activities and found some enjoyment from occupational therapy. She never knew when to come for her medication and needed encouragement with her diet. The kardex was of limited value as it was mainly composed of statements such as 'co-operative' and 'helpful' which conveyed little information as to her progress.

Occupational therapist's report

The occupational therapist said that Mrs X was incapable of shopping though she could cook fairly well. She was still proficient at such tasks as housework and talked enthusiastically about gardening.

Social work report
There was no social work report on this particular patient. A hospital social worker had visited Mrs X to make sure he could visit and was taking care of himself but no formal report had been written.

G.P.'s report
In conversation with the patient's G.P. he said that he had little contact with Mrs X but regular monthly appointments with Mrs X at the surgery for his anti-Parkinson medication. The G.P. was happy to let the community psychiatric nurse visit Mrs X after discharge as long as he was informed of any changes in medication or the mental state of Mrs X.

Community psychiatric nurse's report of patient's initial interview
'The first time Mrs X was interviewed she presented as a rather frightened but apparently physically active person. She viewed me with obvious suspicion and asked what I wanted. I explained that before long she would be going out of hospital and I would be coming to see her at home. She expressed some fear of this and was very concerned that she did not understand her tablets and when to take them. She was also unhappy about the pressures her return home would put on her husband. I tried to put her a little more at ease by asking her to tell me a little bit about herself, her family, her husband and her life at home. She proved an admirable historian and with her information I gained a picture of the following background:
Mrs X was now 69 years old and her husband two years younger. She had not known her father very well although she knew he was a wheelwright and drank rather heavily. He died at the age of 51 of bronchitis. Her mother was very close to Mrs X and they have lived together until Mrs X had got married at the age of 45. Her mother died the following year at the age of 75. Mrs X had two younger sisters; one had died (she did not know what from) and the other lived in London. She said the remaining sister had little contact with her and they did not 'get on'. Mrs X married her husband 'for company' and they had always been happy together. She had decided she was too old to have children and they rarely had sexual intercourse but enjoyed a close relationship. They had spent many happy holidays together on the continent but, starting eight years previously she had got 'fed up', and they rarely went on holiday again. She felt the neighbours were snooty and were interfering with her life. She showed signs of feeling inferior to them. She was also very concerned for the safety of her husband.

She told me he had an illness which, when she told me the symptoms, I recognised to be Parkinson's disease. She did not know why she had been admitted but thought it was good to 'have a rest'.

Her non-verbal behaviour indicated suspicion, mistrust, anxiety and agitation. There were various ways she communicated this; through her gestures, hand-wringing and seated posture. Her mode of dress indicated some difficulty with colour choice, and she was slightly untidy, although overall appearance was socially acceptable.'

Husband's interview
'Mr X was a very pleasant man and made me feel particularly welcome in his home. He was only too pleased to see someone who, he thought, could help him get his wife back home again, and he told me the history leading up to the present events.

He corroborated his wife's history but gave a different slant on the events preceding her admission. He said his wife had stopped working as soon as they got married and eventually they bought the house they were now living in, a pleasant semi-detached in a cul-de-sac. When they moved in, the houses were all new and they had made friends with all the neighbours without difficulty. All went well for the first eight years; then new neighbours began to arrive. They were all young newly-weds and had little in common with Mr and Mrs X. Mrs X began to feel inferior, out of touch and was rude to the neighbours and their children. This of course hardly improved relationships and the neighbours began to leave them alone. Then, about six years ago, Mrs X had begun to say to him that people had been in the house and she hung large heavy curtains at the windows to stop them 'looking in'. Mr X endeavoured to keep some sort of relationship going with the neighbours and succeeded only marginally. It was at this time that Mrs X had also stopped going on holiday and become more and more isolated. She refused to go out shopping and he was virtually running the house. About three years ago he was told he had Parkinson's disease. He was put on chemotherapy which had helped to some extent and retired from his salesman/buyer job six months prematurely. Although he had quite marked limb rigidity and loss of locomotor function, he could still do the shopping and look after himself with a little help.

The house was obviously tidy and Mr X was coping well with living on his own. He indicated that he was an efficient and economical shopper but his cooking ability was limited. His non-verbal behaviour indicated that he was a warm and very friendly person. He showed an obvious delight in being able to talk to someone and said I should call whenever I wished.'

Nursing care plan

Problem A: Medication	Nursing Intervention
Need for regular doses of prescribed medication and observation for side effects *Goal:* Family self-sufficiency in taking of all medication except modecate	1. 'tablet taking' chart drawn up for husband and wife's medication 2. Husband instructed and put in charge of medication 3. Community Psychiatric nurse to administer 2/52 modecate injection. 4. Community psychiatric nurse to observe for side effects of phenothiazines 5. General practitioner asked not to alter medication without notifying community psychiatric nurse

Problem B: Diet	Nursing intervention
1. Need for an adequate and balanced dietary intake	a. Task division between husband and wife: *Husband* *Wife* shopping cooking b. Hospital dietician asked for a balanced and easy to follow diet plan. Husband and wife instructed on how to follow plan
2. Physical inability to eat solid food *Goal:* Regular and sufficient dietary intake	a. Dental consultation sought to check on patient's gross dental caries and infected gums b. Soft diet initiated until this is rectified

Problem C: Caring agencies communication	Nursing intervention
1. Consultant, general practitioner and community psychiatric nurse all providing different care *Goal:* Good patient coverage. Adequate interdisciplinary communication with the community psychiatric nurse acting as co-ordinator	1. Two monthly psychiatric out-patient appointments made 2. 2/52 communication with general practitioner, organised or as necessary 3. Community psychiatric nurse to visit each day for the first week then every three days for three weeks, then once weekly

Problem D: Resocialisation	*Nursing intervention*
1. Patient does not communicate with anyone except husband and community psychiatric nurse	1.
	a. Introduce husband to social club one night per week
	b. Invite patient and husband on outing and trips organised by community psychiatric staff
Goal: Widen friendship group, re-establish old friendships. Re-organise introverted life style	c. Encourage letter writing to old friends
2. Patient will not leave the house as she thinks people will look at her and ridicule her	2. Commence simple progressive desensitisation programme
	a. Walk to end of road with student nurse
Goal: Re-establish friendship with neighbours by 'being seen' and widen social horizons	b. Walk to shops with student nurse
	c. Go shopping with husband
	d. Acknowledge neighbours with simple 'good mornings' etc
	e. Gardening activities encouraged
3. Patient fears she is putting too much pressure on her husband but dare not tell him her fears	3. Encourage two-way communication between husband and wife. Community psychiatric nurse to act as a catalyst initially
Goal: Re-establish communication betwen patient and husband	

Care plan to be evaluated in one month's time

Care plan evaluation after one month

Problem A: Effective medication established and maintained.

Problem B: Task division worked well but patient refuses to go to the dentist. *Goal re-set:* Dental consultant re-set for four weeks' time when patient more reassured.

Problem C: Good communication established between caring agencies. Visits re-adjusted to twice weekly (review in month).

Problem D:

1. Patient and husband attending the social club but Mrs X refuses to go on a day trip. Has written one letter to her sister.

2. 'Desensitisation programme' completed in three sessions but Mrs X will not acknowledge her neighbours. *Goal re-set:* investigate with social and recreational nurse the possibility of a more constructed social skills retraining plan.

3. Some progress in communication but still requires catalyst action by the community psychiatric nurse.

Case study B

A telephone message is received by a community psychiatric nurse from a local general practitioner to say that he has problems with a lady who repeatedly turns up at his surgery asking for help as she is 'run down'. The general practitioner cannot identify any overt depressive symptoms. Can the community psychiatric nurse see her and offer any advice?

Community psychiatric nurse's initial interview at home

'Miss B lives alone in a detached house in a rural area. She is 59 years old, single and with no living relative. The house is neat and clean, the garden well kept.

Miss B was a little surprised at being visited by anyone and did not expect anyone to call although arrangements had been made through the general practitioner. After initial greetings and introductions I explained that the general practitioner had thought I might be of some assistance as Miss B was feeling 'run down' and had visited the general practitioner six times in the last four weeks without any resolution to the symptoms of which she complained. Miss B offered me tea and gave me a description of the symptoms of feeling run down, these were:

1. listlessness;
2. constipation;
3. boredom;
4. occasional feelings of anxiety;
5. loneliness.

I asked her to enlarge on her 'loneliness' and the following history emerged. Miss B is an only child, she and her mother had lived together all her life. She was a shop assistant until three years ago when she had left her work to look after her ailing mother. Two years later her mother died. Her father had been killed in the First World War and she had never known him. She described her relationship with her mother as close and loving; they had experienced no quarrels or major upsets and had led a quiet and ordinary life. She had never married but 'came close to it once'; she had men friends who occasionally took her out but it had always been 'platonic'.

She described the last year of her mother's life as 'heavy going' and she had nursed her mother quite intensively over the last three months of her life.

I asked how she felt when her mother died and she described it as feeling an emptiness but she said she had not shed any tears 'when she went' as it had been a 'bit of a relief'. She had become 'run down' shortly after her mother's death and had been out very little since then. She then wanted to know if tablets were available to help her and if I could get her something as the other tablets were no good and she had stopped taking them after five days.

Her non-verbal behaviour indicated anxiety and this increased when she spoke of her mother. She maintained some eye contact but this was lost when her anxiety increased.

The only other source of information for the case was from the local general practitioner who was new to the area and did not know the patient very well. He had given her some anxiolytic medication to relieve the anxiety she complained of, but with little effect.'

Nursing care plan

Problem A: Medication	Nursing intervention
Looking for tablets to 'cure' her problems when they do not 'work'. Patient discontinues taking the medication *Goal:* Regular anxiolytic medication	1. Explain the need for sustained regular medication 2. Explain and reassure about the purpose of the medication 3. Community psychiatric nurse to observe for side-effects of medication

Problem B: Visits to G.P.'s surgery	Nursing intervention
Visiting general practitioner for reassurance and new medication two to three times per week *Goal:* Relationship formation with community psychiatric nurse	1. Community psychiatric nurse to visit patient once per week at home 2. General practitioner to be informed of plan and kept up to date on progress 3. Patient asked not to go to the general practitioner's surgery without letting the community psychiatric nurse know first 4. Patient given a telephone number where a message can be left for the community psychiatric nurse

Problem C: Unresolved grief reaction	Nursing intervention
Patient unable to come to terms with her feelings now her mother is dead *Goal:* Resolution of guilt feelings and encouragement of coping mechanism	1. Establish a working relationship with the patient 2. Institute grief counselling
Patient is isolating herself from old friends and relationships *Goal:* Re-establish old friendships and get patient to attend social group	1. Encourage the contacting of old friends 2. Introduce patient to a local social group 3. Encourage to go out

Care plan to be evaluated at six weeks

Care plan evaluation at six weeks

Problem A: Regular medication maintained. Anxiolytic medication cut by half after consultation with the general practitioner.

Problem B: Patient has not been back to the doctors surgery. Uses the telephone number on occasions to 'test' the community psychiatric nurse. Visits can now be cut to once a fortnight.

Problem C: Working relationship established with the patient. Patient is working through her feelings fairly well, some friends have rallied round after she had contacted them. Patient has attended the social club, but does not like it. *Goal re-set:* No further encouragement regarding the social club as the friends have compensated for this.

PREVENTIVE PSYCHIATRY AND PREVENTIVE PSYCHIATRIC NURSING

The traditional approach to psychiatry is one of 'cure' and most of the available services are based on this model. It requires someone to be 'ill' and then 'treatment' to be given where appropriate. This treatment is aimed nowadays at fast results in terms of short stay care and intensive treatment.

It is possible to take a different approach and instead of curing, aim some of our efforts at preventing illness. This is not a new argument. It has long been the approach used in public health and is an integral part of the work of the health visitors and occupational health nurses. It should also be part of the total role of the community psychiatric nurse.

There are few other authors who have laid out this approach as clearly as Gerald Caplan in his two books *Principles of Preventive Psychiatry* and *An Approach to Community Mental Health* (both Tavistock Publications).

What is preventive psychiatry?

Preventive psychiatry attempts to do a number of things. It changes emphasis from the cure of the mentally ill to the maintainance of the mentally well which means that it seeks to identify those things which cause or contribute towards mental illness and stop them causing illness or at least minimise the impact by softening their effects on potential victims. There are three main areas within preventive psychiatry: primary, secondary and tertiary, and within each of these three areas we can look at methods of intervention in two ways. These are on an individualistic level and looking at the community as a whole.

Primary prevention

Primary prevention aims to reduce the chances of people becoming mentally ill. As we do not know the exact causes of mental illness it could be argued that this is an unreasonable area to aim at. There are, however, definite indications pointing towards factors which can precipitate and contribute towards mental illness and it is possible to exert influence over these factors. Public health programmes worked along these lines in their early days. The great Victorian health reformers did not know the exact causes of disease and ill health but aimed towards eradicating known associated factors with great success.

Secondary prevention

Secondary prevention seeks to minimise the effects of established mental disorder. The people involved in this area will already have the early signs and symptoms of mental disorder, but by finding them very early on in their illness and by bringing swift and effective care to their aid, it is possible to reduce the duration and severity of the illness considerably.

Tertiary prevention

This is familiar to most psychiatric nurses. Tertiary prevention seeks to reduce the residual effects of mental disorder and the disabilities which it leaves. These are the positive rehabilitation aspects of aftercare which most areas now practice to some extent.

Where can the community psychiatric nurse get involved?

As mentioned earlier there are two main approaches to preventive care; the individualistic approach, and working with the community as a whole; and there are openings in both areas for the community psychiatric nurse to work in.

Health education

Health education has application in all areas of preventive psychiatry. Primary health education concerns itself totally with the healthy and not with the sick. Working in this area presents some difficulty as the foundations of good mental health are laid down very early in life, which means that for most people it is their dynamics of family life which are all important. It can therefore be stated that those things which are essential to satisfactory and happy family life should be encouraged and those which are antagonistic should be changed. Some of these factors are already approached on a community wide basis by other professionals such as health visitors. National bodies exist for the promotion of health education i.e. The Health Education Council.

The essentials of family psychiatry and associated research are outlined in considerable detail by J. G. Howells(4). Given insights into the background of family interactions and influences, the community psychiatric nurse should be able to work out areas where they could work in primary health education.

Health education in secondary prevention is involved in the education of the lay person and other professionals about the early detection of mental disorders. In secondary health education the disorder will already have established itself, but early detection will reduce its effects. The people most likely to notice the onset of mental disorders are not the professional agencies of the general practitioner, the psychiatrist or the social worker, but the relations and friends of the potential victim. By educating the general public about the early signs and symptoms of mental disorder, it is possible they will refer their friends and relatives earlier for prompt and effective treatment. There are hidden dangers for the inexperienced health educator, false impressions about the nature and effects of mental disorder and sensationalism for the sake of impact should be avoided at all costs as this often perpetuates the fear of mental illness and may prevent people from seeking help.

Health education involved in tertiary care has implications for the community psychiatric nurses working with the rehabilitation and return of the mentally ill in the community. There is a need to educate these people who have already been ill about the possibility of recurring symptoms and what indications they should watch out for. Also, where people are living, for example, in the group home setting there may be local opposition to the siting of a 'home for the mentally ill'. There is, in such a situation, an obvious area where the community psychiatric nurse can work in reducing prejudice and stigma.

Examples of broad areas for health education are:

1. Physical health and its relationship to mental disorder.
2. Signs and symptoms of mental disorder.
3. Relations 'self-help programmes'.
4. Instruction of and discussion with other professionals.

Health education is not popular with those people who need to justify results in terms of numbers and statistical proof, as the results are difficult to measure in terms of prevented admissions or drop in illness levels, so the expense is, perhaps, difficult to justify but it has proved its worth in general medicine. Health education should form an integral part of the total role of the community psychiatric nurse and although perhaps practised at a rudimentary level in some areas community psychiatric nurses need to examine the resources available and the techniques of basic teaching which can improve their performance in the teaching situation.

Screening systems for identifying mental illness

If we are aware of some of the early signs and symptoms of mental illness, what are the chances of improving secondary prevention by identifying these people who are already on the verge of illness or in the early stages, from the healthy members of the community? Screening is one way of doing this.

There are a variety of screening programmes which can be considered and which have proved their worth in general medicine. Mass radiography, breast clinics and cytological smear clinics have all been used to find the early stages of physical illness with marked success. While psychiatry has been a little slower to catch on to this area there are now a number of studies in operation which use the common principles applied to screening.

This section will outline the principles applied to screening and show some of the problems in applying these principles to mental disorder.

To take a screening test to the population demands that those running the screening service find a 'captive' population. It would not be practical to go on to the streets and present questions to people walking by. Screening demands that captive groups are accessible, willing to co-operate and are easily traced in case of the discovering of potential mental disorder. Examples of such groups are; attenders to a general practitioner's surgery, industry and educational establishments. The screeners also need to assume that the 'captive' group is willing to participate and, if identified, be willing to be treated. Having discovered the captive group, the screening can be done either by interview or by a questionnaire which is filled in by the participant. Once a number of these have been done it is then possible to 'weed out' the potential victims and provide prompt and effective treatment, this is secondary prevention at its best.

There are a number of schemes in operation at the moment. Experimental sample surveys have been tried and published, for example: Johnstone and Goldberg(5) and Pike(6). Both these studies have implications for those working in the community, Johnstone and Goldberg describe the 'value of the screening procedure in the secondary prevention of psychiatric disorders', Pike, in his study describes people who have not contacted their doctor for some time and who may have unreported illness or social problems, 'These problems if left undetected may lead to medical or social breakdown compelling admission to welfare homes or hospital'.

There is some evidence to show that screening has a considerable part to play in effective secondary care. Even a simple questionnaire on physical well-being may turn up people, especially the elderly who may be otherwise seen later on suffering from depression or anxiety. The community psychiatric nurse should be aware of the tool of screening and possibly be involved in associated programmes.

CRISIS INTERVENTION

Crisis intervention has become a term often quoted by community psychiatric nurses as part of their role, but on closer examination most of the work performed by community psychiatric nurses in this area is done following a crisis. This means that, strictly speaking, it is not intervention and it could be better referred to as just crisis work. This section will outline some of the theories behind crisis intervention and then examine by case study two ways in which crisis intervention can help in preventive psychiatry.

Crisis theory
There are different approaches to crisis theory, from the broader views (Brandon, 7) to the idea that the foundations of theory are firmly based in ego-psychology (Caplan, 8). The concept of crisis theory and crisis intervention has had its champions for a long time within social work and there are a variety of documented studies (Parad, 9) but is not well known within the nursing and medical professions.

Crisis theory, broadly speaking, implies that within us all there are 'coping mechanisms' which we use to deal with the problems and crises which life presents to us. These mechanisms are supported by sets of values, problem-solving skills and powers of perception. The level of their development will depend to a large extent upon the cultural influences and stability of the person's environment. One of the consequences of this is that a crisis to some people will be no more than a ripple to others. An individual's personal experiences in dealing with problems in the past will also provide some measure of ability to deal with a problem in the future. Problems which in the past have been resolved by such measures as rationalisation, regression or repression doubtless affect the way people deal with a new problem which has similarities to those previously resolved in this way. It could well be, however, that a new crisis presents a person with an insurmountable problem, and although they have resolved crises in the past quite adequately, they find the current problem impossible to tackle. When this threatening situation is realised as being not easily resolved then a state of crisis is developing and this produces vague feelings of discomfort and tension. From this state there is a movement into feelings of anxiety or shame or guilt and the person becomes more helpless than usual and often quite disorganised. There are therefore two alternatives open when faced with crises. It is possible to resolve the crisis using past experiences and, having resolved the crisis in a new way, become an even more coping person because of it. Secondly we can collapse into disorganisation when faced with crises and it is at this time that mental disorder may result.

There are stages in everyone's life when crisis is a higher risk than at other times, such as adolscence, change of job, marriage, having a child or retirement. At all these times the stress factors are changed and present a new experience with which people have to cope. If there is an indication that people are not going to cope, then that is the right time for crisis intervention, during the crisis peak or before that, rather than when a person has sought refuge in an unhealthy coping mechanism or mental disorder.

The progression of crises has been documented in a number of studies by Lindemanne(10), Bowlby, Ainsworth, Boston, and Rosenbluth(11), and Decker and Stubblebine(12).

In the following case studies it is possible to identify the timing and results of intervention.

Case study A

Mrs B, aged 59, lived with her daughter and son-in-law, Mr and Mrs S, and their two children for two years. They had a three-bedroomed house and two rooms downstairs, conditions were adequate but a little strained as all rooms in the house were small. Mrs B had been diagnosed as schizophrenic and she had had three admissions to hospital, the last occasion being some two years previously. After one discharge she had been given a council flat but found it too big to cope with and had eventually been given a smaller flat. She expressed dissatisfaction with this as she did not like the neighbours. After one more unsuccessful move to a similar flat she had to be re-admitted to hospital.

On the next discharge she expressed a wish to live with her daughter and son-in-law as they had enough room and were willing to take her. Mr S telephoned the community psychiatric nurse to say that he was worried about Mrs B as she was showing signs of her 'old illness' coming back again. The community psychiatric nurse visited them at home and after discussions with all concerned found that there was considerable anxiety and tension on all sides, which had arisen when Mrs S had written to the local authorities asking for a larger house as the children were growing up and needed separate rooms. The authorities had replied that there was a waiting list for larger houses but they could re-locate Mrs B in a flat temporarily. Mr S had discussed this with Mrs B but she was unwilling to do this. The community psychiatric nurse identified the following problems:

Mrs B
Previous experiences:
1. Unable to cope with living on her own.
2. A need for the immediate security of having her family around her.

Presenting crises:
1. Having to move back into a situation where she did not previously cope, thereby invoking old fears and anxieties.
2. Loss of immediate contact with family.
3. Guilt feelings about being 'in the way' and not helping in the current situation.

Mr & Mrs S
Previous experiences:
1. Mrs B becomes 'ill' when pressured.
2. Mrs B cannot manage on her own.

Presenting crises:
1. Need for more room for the children.
2. Inability to move.
3. Guilt feelings about 'pushing' mother out and precipitating another 'illness' episode.

Resolution of crises
The community psychiatric nurse undertook the following tasks in order to prevent the crises producing major upset:
1. Letters from a general practitioner and social work report were sent to the local authorities asking for priority to be given to Mr S's case. This was duly given.
2. The community psychiatric nurse acted as a therapeutic 'catalyst' so that everyone knew how everyone else was feeling in the current situation.
3. The community psychiatric nurse monitored Mrs B's response to the crisis and by supportive visits and temporary

adjustment of her medication prevented re-admission to hospital.

Case study B

Mr T was a 22-year-old single man who was waiting for corrective orthopaedic surgery to a congenitally deformed left hand. He had been placed on a 'cold' surgery list on two occasions and on each occasion had not gone for surgery on the pretext of some other illness. He now had to go for a third time and the general practitioner asked the community psychiatric nurse to 'have a word' as he was known to be an anxious and difficult man and it was thought that perhaps that he would not attend this time either. The community psychiatric nurse interviewed the man at the surgery and the following points emerged. Mr T had been into hospital as a child on three separate occasions and he said that on each occasion he had been very frightened and that he did not want 'to go through all that again'. Mr T also said that the current operation was not essential and yet he displayed a lot of self-consciousness about his deformity and as a consequence there was a lot of contradictory information about his true feelings on the matter. He stated that it was his parents who wanted him to have the operation; then later on he said that the deformity interfered with his social life and 'turned the girls off'.

Mr T
Previous experiences:
1. Traumatic experiences of hospital as a child.
2. Resolution of previous appointments by sublimation by using other illnesses.
3. His deformity interfered with his social life.

Presenting crises:
1. Hospitalisation—re-awakening of old fears.
2. Anticipatory worry about the operation.
3. Contradictory feelings about the benefits of surgery and the possibility of pain and discomfort.

Resolution of crises
1. Mr T was given supportive psychotherapy about his fears on the subject of hospitalisation and surgery.
2. Mr T was offered a visit to the orthopaedic ward to see how modern and comfortable it was.

It has already been mentioned that it is possible to identify areas in everyone's life where a potential crisis may occur. Using the previously outlined technique of health education it is possible to alert the community to the hazards which these events may provoke, and also to provide some counter measures to their effects.

Such areas as:

1. pre-retirement instruction classes,
2. pre-marriage advice and guidance,
3. pre-natal classes,

already exist in most areas and are provided not by psychiatric services but by such diverse 'disciplines' as the clergy, midwifery staff and the general public: so there is no necessity for the intrusion of psychiatry into these areas. However, an awareness of the concepts of crisis theory and intervention should be borne in mind when providing a community psychiatric nursing service.

REFERENCES

1. Daubenmire, M. J. and King, I. M. (1973) Nursing process models: a systems approach, *Nursing Outlook*, **21**, No. 8, 512–17.
2. Orlando, I. D. (1961) *The Dynamic Nurse and Patient Relationship.* New York: G. P. Putman and Sons.
3. Mayers, M. G. (1972) *A Systematic Approach to the Nursing Care Plan.* New York: Appleton-Century-Croft.
4. Howells, J. G. *Theory and Practice of Family Psychiatry.* London: Oliver and Boyd.
5. Johnstone, A. and Goldberg, D. (1976) Psychiatric screening in general practice, *Lancet*, March 20, 605–608.
6. Pike, L. A. (1976) Screening the elderly in general practice, *Journal of the Royal College of General Practitioners*, 2,698–703.
7. Brandon, S. (1970) Crisis theory and possibilities of crisis intervention, *British Journal of Psychiatry*, 117, No. 541, 000.
8. Caplan, G. (1964) *Principles of Preventive Psychiatry.* London: Tavistock Publications.
9. Parad, H. J. (1965) *Crisis Intervention: Selected Readings.* New York: Family Service Association of America.
10. Lindemanne, E. (1948) Symptomatology and management of acute grief, *American Journal of Psychiatry*, 101, 141–48.
11. Bowlby, J., Ainsworth, M., Boston, M. and Rosenbluth, Dd. (1956) The effects of mother-child separation—a follow up study, *British Journal of Medical Psychology*, 79, 211–47.
12. Decker, B. J. and Stubblebine, M. D. (1972) Crisis intervention and prevention of psychiatric disability—a follow up study, *American Journal of Psychiatry*, 129:6, 000

SUGGESTIONS FOR FURTHER READING

Caplan, G. (1964) *Principles of Preventive Psychiatry.* London: Tavistock
Caplan, G. (1974) *An Approach to Community Mental Health.* London: Tavistock
Hart, C. E. (1975) *Screening in General Practice.* Edinburgh: Churchill Livingstone.
Little, D. E. and Carnevali, D. L. (1976) *Nursing Care Planning.* Philadelphia: J. B. Lippincott Co.
Berni, R. and Fordyce, W. E. (1973) *Behavior Modification and the Nursing Process.* St. Louis: Mosby Co.

Goldman, E. (ed.) (1972) *Community Mental Health Nursing*. New York: Appleton Century Crofts.

Grace, H. K., Layton, J. and Camilleri, D. (1977) *Mental Health Nursing. A Socio-Psychological Approach*. Dubuque, Iowa: Wm. C. Brown Co.

Caplan, G. (1970) *The Theory and Practice of Mental Health Consultation*. London: Tavistock.

6

Strategies for care in community mental handicap nursing

The community team in mental handicap is very much in its infancy; many teams are in the developmental stage at present and not fully engaged in providing a service for families. What the nurse does varies from one authority to another. What the nurse could and should do elicits different answers from different people depending on the basic philosophy regarding the functions of the nurse of the mentally handicapped—the arguments being extended from the hospital to the community—and to some extent depends on the concept of 'community care' adopted.

Community care can mean all the services provided outside the hospital; it can mean the use of resources and services within the community; the term is applied to handicapped people who are living outside of hospital but not necessarily receiving services, and community care can be care given in a locality by friends, relatives and neighbours. There have been a number of unfortunate experiences, the more so because the results should have been forseen, in which patients have been discharged to live in seaside hotels and establishments intended for a more transient population, spending their empty time aimlessly wandering the streets. This may be loosely regarded as care in the community but it is not community care. The same would apply to discharged residents who for one reason or another fail to become integrated into a community, either because of community or personal factors, resulting in isolation and withdrawal such that residential care may be preferable.

Many people with a variety of handicapping conditions are maintained at home by family, friends and neighbours, more perhaps than are so maintained by recognised agencies. The community nurse should supplement rather than supplant the caring already in existence and to this end should help to co-ordinate and encourage assistance from the immediate vicinity rather then mobilising 'foreign' forces from outside the immediate neighbourhood. The research on the help families receive is conflicting. D. Wilkin found that many families received little or no help from family and friends (see M. Bayley).

The community nurse will have some overlap of role with the health visitor, school nurse and the social worker, and it is important that the family is not over-visited or given conflicting advice. The provision of a laundry or incontinence service by one agency may interfere with the toilet training programme being set up by another. Finding a niche in areas where other professionals are already engaged and have been so for some time, causes some consternation. The person to visit should be the best person available for the particular situation. A great deal of liaison and co-operation will thus be involved.

The base for the nurse will depend on the concept of community care, whether the hospital is seen as apart from or as part of the community. Many services are originating from the hospital as might be expected. The arguments for their continuance from this base include access to beds, access to other professionals e.g. physio-therapists, language therapists, psychologists and psychiatrists. If the hospital is a resource centre to the community it serves, a nurse whose operational base is outside the hospital should have these services available and have access to the wider resources of other specialist units, multiple handicap units, paediatric and communication centres and perchance being based outside the hospital develop a more family/client orientation than otherwise. The nurse should be aware of all the services, local and national, statutory and voluntary, that are available and should maintain a close liaison with those agencies helpful to herself and her client. These would include day facilities provided by education, family and community or social services as well as the residential services including the hospital.

The community nurse must be aware of the developments within the health service, as well as the community service, maintaining close links with the residential establishments that are available for short term and emergency use in order that clients may be appropriately placed. Continuity of care is one of the myths of nursing, yet it would be preferable to have those responsible for residential care at the caring inter-face to be involved with the client to some degree in the home and in the hostel or hospital as part of the pre-admission, post-discharge or follow-up procedure in order that the residential team are aware of the total needs of the client and/or his family. This is not to advocate a ward-based community service. Some hospitals do, however, use nurses from wards or community based hostels to execute some of the functions it is appropriate to call community nursing. The degree to which such nurses can be involved with liaising between agencies, and providing a service to families, and to efficiently manage the residential establishment as well, requires fine balancing if the specialised areas of hospital and residential care, whose efficient functioning is vital to a comprehensive service, are not to be less efficiently managed than they might otherwise be. The involvement of the residential team should be the responsibility, and come under the direction of, a full time community nurse. The residential and non-residential are elements of the same service, neither being superior to the other. The aim is the production of a united comprehensive service to the handicapped and their families, not to create a divisive and potentially elitist group of nurses.

By being aware of the total service available to the mentally handicapped, the community nurse acts as a catalyst unifying the service around the client, reducing the gaps between professionals and especially between the long established hospitals and the community services.

Gaining acceptance for the community nurse for the mentally handicapped has not always been easy. Another community worker can be expected to cause concern amongst professionals already working with the family. However, once the expertise of the mental handicap nurse is appreciated, largely through the pioneering efforts of the nurses (initially working alone, who have made it a priority to inform all people whom it concerned of their particular area of expertise and the service they intend to give), these nurses have not only been accepted but welcomed as valuable colleagues. As the nurse should be supplementing, not supplanting, the work of the family, so it is with the professionals. The nurse adds her specialist knowledge and skills to the community pool. Although an overlapping of respon-sibilities with other professionals is likely, as each appreciates the role of the other, the common boundaries will be established between individual workers in order that the family receives a comprehensive and unified service fitting the perceived needs.

ASSESSMENT AS A BASIS OF CARE

A comprehensive assessment of the needs of the client and family must be obtained involving the nurse and the family. Assessment (like community care) has become a much abused term, it is not an end in itself but must lead to action. In the preparation of care programmes and ongoing training programmes for both client and family it is essential to accurately observe and record a base line of circumstances and behaviour with the active participation of the family. Too often in the past the parents have been excluded from the process of care which has itself been largely based on intuition and guesswork. Separate consideration must be given to the needs of the client and those of the family, and a balance between those needs maintained.

When considering the needs of the handicapped the three strands of (1) difficulty in learning, (2) developmental delay, and (3) socially imposed handicap, needs to be borne in mind. To what extent are the difficulties encountered due to features inherent in the condition and to what extent manifest through management or caring relationships? Comprehensive assessment may involve attendance at a day-centre or even a period as an in-patient. The latter is not to be encouraged for the sake of expediency, as the disturbance to the client may not only give an inaccurate assessment, but have a detrimental effect on the person and his relationships with others. Cases will arise, however, when an in-patient placement is the only way a satisfactory assessment can be made.

At the day centre for children the paediatrician, paediatric nurses, physiotherapist, speech and occupational therapists, teachers and psychologist will independently carry out their own assessment procedures reporting back to a case-conference at which the future caring strategy will be determined. Teachers in the special schools execute their own assessment on which their individual teaching is based, assessment being an integral part of teaching.

For the mentally handicapped adult the picture is a little different. Some areas now have assessment units for adults attending the training centres in order that a programme may be devised to match the needs of the client, to extend his social skills, range of coping techniques and continue his further education, rather than to meet the needs of the training centre (especially those that have yet to lose their preoccupation with output—the 2000 by Friday syndrome). These assessments take place over weeks or months producing as a result a detailed balanced training and educational programme.

The combination of the length of the assessment, the time on the waiting list for assessment and the preceding time before some one decides that an assessment is necessary, results in a relatively small number of people who are adequately assessed leaving many who require programmes of care to be implemented before such a comprehensive assessment can be carried out. It is therefore essential that the community nurse is prepared to carry out discreet observation assessment and recording in the home. What is more—the parents should be involved in the assessment and encouraged to use the assessment tool themselves in the production of training programmes.

A number of different forms of assessment are in use, some more commonly than others. Although subject to developmental delay the mentally handicapped substantially go through the same sequence of

child development as the non-handicapped child. Ordinary developmental scales may thus be used to determine the stage in the sequence
that the child has reached on any given criteria—play, social
development, speech, sensory and motor skills, emotional adjustment—which will give a developmental profile. This can then be used
as a baseline on which to produce a programme in order to encourage
and promote progress to the next stage in the developmental sequence.
Reference need not be made to the normal age at which any criterion is
reached but to use the information to set target behaviour in the
sequence of development for which the programme is devised.

The 'Portage system' developed in Wisconsin in the U.S.A. is an
assessment procedure based on child development information.
Having obtained a base-line this system contains a prescriptive
element, the number indicating the level attained in the respective area
of performance directs the content and method to be used to facilitate
progress to the subsequent stage in the five areas of language, motor,
cognitive, socialisation and self-help.

This eliminates the tedious task of devising the programme, a task
not beyond the skilled teacher and is thus a great time saver. The
system has the disadvantage of being American requiring modification
in some items for English children, it has however, the very real
advantage that information about a child's level of attainment and a
prescriptive programme can easily be transmitted to interested parties
by the simple expedient of listing the relevant numbers in a letter,
card-file or case notes. The receiving teacher, nursery or community
nurse providing they have access to the Portage box of numbered cards
can follow the same programme instructing the parents in the same.
This obviates the necessity for lengthy individual training programmes which are of the essence short lived.

There are numerous scales of social maturity, social competence,
independence, adaptive behaviour and functional behaviour of which
the best known are in all probability the progress assessment charts
(P.A.C.) devised by H. C. Gunzburg. The visual display of these
charts is particularly useful, readily illustrating not only progress in
the respective areas but also any imbalance in performance which may
need correction. This is shown by the discrepancy between
communication and fine motor skills compared with self-help and
gross motor skills arising from the relative amount of practice rather
than lack of inate ability. Some practitioners have found the steps
between the criteria on the P.A.C. chart to be too large for some
clients, a finer gradation being required. Once competence in the
techniques of assessment is mastered the possibility of individual
teams developing their own *ad hoc* scales arises. These may fall short

on transferability but will be a more useful therapeutic tool than inappropriate commercial scales of doubtful value.

Assessment is not an end in itself but must lead to action. Consciously or not the nurse makes assumptions about the care any given patient/client requires using a combination of previous knowledge, experience, intuition and guesswork, the 'finger in the wind' philosophy. Some nurses are inherently more capable of making sound judgements than others about the service and care required. These nurses give an excellent service to the client without seriously considering assessment or caring strategies; the nursing process as a basis is unknown to them. A systematised assessment format removes the chance element from care enabling the less gifted to have a sound basis on which to prepare a care-plan. A balance between the competing needs of the client on the limited time of the family and his all round development can be achieved.

Whatever system the nurse uses for assessment purposes, it is important that they have an accurate, unambiguous assessment on sound criteria and adequately recorded.

Goal planning

As the nursing of the mentally handicapped has moved away from the medical model of care, away from the psychodynamic, physiological, genetic and social press theories of explaining retarded behaviour, it has moved towards seeking the determinants of behaviour in learning theory, adopting a behavioural approach. One of the many advantages of this approach, exemplified in the nursing process, is the shift of the locus from the client to the 'teacher'. From a base-line of assessment criteria the needs of the client are placed in hierarchical order in terms of importance to the client. A goal is then selected and described in clear unequivocal behavioural terms. This objective should be one that it is possible to obtain in a short space of time, days rather than weeks. A care plan is then devised and implemented with due consideration to the content and method of the instruction. The final stage concerns evaluation of the care plan and its effectiveness in attaining the objective and satisfying the perceived need. The evaluation is of the care plan, the effectiveness of the teaching, not that of the learning. This helps towards a situation where consideration is given not to what a person can do but the more positive approach of how much help and of what kind he needs to complete a task.

Goal planning, using realistic achievable goals in a strict time limit described in concrete terms, is the basis of teaching the mentally handicapped. It is the ability to reduce everyday skills to extremely small steps whether it be tying a shoe-lace, operating a zip, or using the toilet, that facilitates the teaching of the mentally handicapped. This can be put to good use by the parents once the basic idea of skill analysis is grasped.

Determining the needs of the family

The needs of the family may be many and varied ranging from advice on day-to-day management, teaching of skills, discipline, support—economic, moral, practical—help with leisure time, domestic aids, home-help, laundry and other services. Whilst one would have no desire to deprive a family of services merely because of the crossing of professional boundaries, it is important that the nurse does not encroach on the province of other professionals unnecessarily.

The family will require support throughout the life-span of their child, at birth if handicap is suspected, at the suspicion of developmental delay, final diagnosis, subsequent family crisis, illness, school placement, adolescence and sexual development, employment, and possible marriage.

The family may need to avail themselves of such services as a playgroup, toy library, nursery, special care facility, special education, day care or short term care. An important function of the community nurse would be in conjunction with others, to mobilise and co-ordinate the available services including the voluntary neighbourhood support services such as they exist; and encouraging their development where they do not, 'sitting' lifting, bathing and transport may all fit this category.

The mother of a normal baby is rarely short of advice as most people feel themselves competent to give it, from the next door neighbour to strangers on the bus. The mother of a handicapped child has, in contrast, a dearth of advice and as a result may embark on strategies that seem right at the time but are inappropriate in the long term. The handicapped child is further handicapped by being treated differently than a 'normal' child to a degree not warranted by his condition. Being often less curious than his fellow—the notorious good baby—the mentally handicapped child is under-stimulated and as a result under-functions. Whilst it is a truism that we can do no better than our genetic make-up will allow, we can—and frequently do—worse. The encouragement of parents to provide an emotionally secure, stimulating environment (bearing in mind the child development sequence of Jean Piaget) is the more important as the moderate, mild and borderline categories of mental retardation (W.H.O. classification of diseases) can be regarded as culturally determined and thus available to corrective measures. The stimulation should be in the areas of sensory-motor and language acquisition. To this end the parents must be encouraged to talk to the child frequently, retaining always an awareness that talking to someone who gives a minimal response is not easy. Use of play group and nursery facilities should be made as well as of toy libraries. The handicapped child, whose progression from one stage to another requires a fine gradation of tasks of increasing difficulty—'small steps for small feet'—cannot make sense of the complicated toys normally purchased for children. Experiencing an incidental learning deficit, the handicapped child requires a structured sequence in order to learn effectively. This would require a large number of toys and similar teaching apparatus with carefully controlled variables, ranging from the very simple to the more complex, in numerous stages. Once the 'toy' had been mastered and the child having progressed to a subsequent stage the toy would be useless to that particular child having little intrinsic value unlike the sophisticated toys to which the normal child returns again and again. A library of toys that can be borrowed at will and returned when their usefulness has been outlived has obvious advantages.

The tendency to allow the handicapped to behave inappropriately is another area where counter-productive caring strategies are adopted. This occurs when the excuse of handicap is used to explain behaviour which would, under normal circumstances, not be tolerated. The child is as a result under-disciplined, invariably leading to difficult behaviour at a later stage and sometimes leading to requests for admission because the person's behaviour cannot be controlled. Early intervention by an experienced practitioner should reduce the strain imposed on a family by the person who behaves differently, making their life more tolerable, and consequently reducing unnecessary admissions to residential care. It must be appreciated that for a minority of families the strain imposed by the presence of a handicapped child will prove intolerable. Suitable residential accommodation to meet the needs of these people should be an essential part of any comprehensive service for the mentally handicapped.

Short term relief

The lack of free time and the limitations on the family's freedom of action are amongst the commonest complaints of the family with a handicapped member. Obtaining a baby sitter is not normally difficult unless the person to be sat with happens to be mentally handicapped and possibly not a child, when 'sitters' are more difficult to come by. This could be an area where local voluntary help could be organised. In many cases, however, the nature of the condition will demand the presence of an experienced person. The presence of a nurse experienced in the care of the handicapped allows mother to visit the hair dressers, the super-market or the out-patient department with confidence. An evening out can once again be a pleasure.

A longer break can be obtained by admission to a suitable unit for day-care, overnight, or for two or three weeks whilst the family have a welcome break, and the opportunity for a holiday. The co-ordination of this type of care which goes under a number of titles—'phased care', 'short term care' and 'programmed care' is a function of the community nurse who should make it their business to be aware of those families who would require such help. Liaison with the voluntary agencies and the local social worker is essential if the maximum use is to be made of this previously under-utilised facility.

Social competence

In order to live in this world it is important that we are aware of the norms and values of the society in which we live and, when appropriate, that we are aware that our behaviour is deviant. This is no less so for the mentally handicapped, and possibly more so. Unable to appreciate rational argument, the mentally handicapped must be taught by example, opportunity and learning, through the strategy of rewarding appropriate behaviour and ignoring inappropriate behaviour, i.e. a 'safe' way of behaving in social situations. The mentally handicapped are much more open, less sophisticated, more naive, more honest, sometimes blunt to the point normally regarded as rude. They are less inhibited, being openly affectionate and often indiscriminately demonstrative. If they are to be accepted the mentally handicapped must not be allowed to behave in a way that will draw attention to their condition. Indiscriminate shouting, talking to strangers, open displays of emotion as well as the more obvious eating, dressing and toileting behaviour, must be maintained within the limits of community tolerance. It is perhaps a cause for sadness that the purity of response of the handicapped has to be so modified, causing one to reflect on the thoughts of the great educator Rousseau, and his thesis that the individual is corrupted by society. Although his work gives the rationale for child-centred learning, it is none-the-less true that if you want to live in this world you must obey the rules.

In training the child the parent can be made aware of the simple strategies of fading of prompt, reverse chaining and the obvious yet inconsistently applied strategy in normal life of rewarding appropriate behaviour and ignoring inappropriate behaviour, securing extinction of the latter by failing to reward it. So often attention-seeking behaviour is learnt by the very fact of notice being taken of it. It needs to be borne in mind that if behaviour exists, something somewhere is reinforcing it. 'Personhood' must be maintained; it would be so easy to produce socially competent robots under the influence of training programmes based on behaviour modification techniques. Social training programmes must co-exist with the developmental training programmes, the handicapped being taught what they are capable of learning and what, for them, is worth learning—hence the insistence on realistic goals based on objective criteria.

Management of leisure

Leisure time is one of the most difficult periods of the day for the growing adolescent and adult to manage.

The filling of free time with meaningful hobbies and pastimes will give the handicapped person not only a fresh interest, but gives a wider range of topics of conversation. Use should be made of such clubs and societies existing in the locality as well as the 'Gateway' club. The activities selected should be in accordance with interests and abilities; the normal childhood pattern of sampling a number of hobbies superficially until an activity that suits ability, personality and pocket becomes apparent. Leisure interests are more often caught than taught. Father particularly should be encouraged to include the child in his own interests. Whilst a hobby is a means of getting away from it all, being in some way involved in care can be so helpful to the child, the family and, especially, the father.

As the profession is developing, changes in attitude are imperative. Nursing is so often seen as doing things for people. We must move to a situation where we are encouraging people to do things for themselves. The nurse must also increasingly think in behavioural terms, formulate short-term objectives, care plans and subsequent evaluation to ascertain the effectiveness of the plan in meeting perceived needs.

The nurse's base must be seen to be the community rather than the hospital and to regard the hospital not as a base or refuge but as a community resource on a par with the other resources available.

FURTHER READING

Bowell, D. M. and Wingrove, J. M. (1974) *The Handicapped Person in the Community*. London: Tavistock Publications.
Bayley, M. (1973) Mental Handicap and Community Care. London: R.K.P.
Clarke, A. M. and Clarke, A. D. B. (1974) *Mental Deficiency – The Changing Outlook*. London: Methuen.
Cunningham, C. and Sloper, P. (1978) *Helping your Handicapped Baby*. London: Souvenir Press (Human Horizon Series).
Fox, M. A. (1975) They get this training but don't really know how you feel, *Action Research for the Crippled Child*. National Foundation for Research into Crippling Diseases.
H.M.S.O. (1975) Mentally handicapped children, *H.M.S.O. Education Pamphlet*, No. 60. London.

Kushlik, A., Felce, D., Palmer, J. and Smith, J. (1976) Evidence to the Committee of Enquiry into Mental Handicap Nursing and care. Winchester (Wessex R.H.A.)

National Development Group (1976) Mental handicap: planning together.

National Development Group (1977a) Mentally handicapped children: A plan of action.

National Development Group (1977b) Day services for mentally handicapped adults.

National Development Group (1977c) Helping mentally handicapped school leavers.

National Development Group (1977d) Residential short-term care for mentally handicapped people: suggestions for action.

Spain, B. and Wigley, G. (1975) *Right from the Start*. London: N.S.M.H.C.C.

Wilkin, D. (1979) Caring for the Mentally Handicapped Child. London: Croom Helm.

Wolfersberger, W. (1967) Counselling parents of the retarded. In *Mental Retardation*, Baumeister, A. (ed). London: London University Press.

7

The behavioural perspective

INTRODUCTION

The behavioural sciences are relatively new as academic disciplines go, having existed as such only since the turn of the century and having been called such since the 1950s.

They need to be distinguished from the social sciences, which formerly encompassed them. They have emerged from under the latter's umbrella to form a reasonably well-defined body of knowledge. This recent venture is at one and the same time less expansive in terms of breadth of knowledge, yet more exhaustive in terms of the depth of knowledge related to human behaviour.

What are the behavioural sciences then? Well, the term was originally intended and is usually understood to indicate the following subject areas:

1. sociology;
2. some anthropology;
3. some psychology, and
4. the behavioural aspects of:
   a. biology;
   b. economics;
   c. geography;
   d. law;
   e. psychiatry, and
   f. political science.
   (cf. Berelson and Steiner(1)).

The question arises as to why this new area of knowledge needed to arise at all when, in fact, all of its subject matter was already encompassed by the social sciences. Some hints of the answer to this question are perhaps already contained in the preceding sentences. What the behavioural sciences promised was not so much the exposition of new areas of knowledge but more the illumining of existing disciplines in respect of all aspects of human behaviour, whether expressed by overt means or implied via attitudes, expectations and so on. This 'approach' necessarily implied the carrying out of a great deal of research based on the rigorous application of methodological principles and was, of course, a long term undertaking. Inherent also in the 'behavioural approach' and a very important component of it was the notion of the interdisciplinary team.

Has the application of the 'behavioural approach' to the social sciences done anything other than create a new term, viz. the behavioural sciences? Well, clearly the very minimum it has achieved has been the focussing of attention on human behaviour as such, through thousands of articles and scores of books (Berelson and Steiner(1)). From the research carried out to enable such articles and books to have been written there has emerged much more:

1. Man, rather than ideologies, rats or trends, has moved to the centre of the stage. Man, being much more capricious and uncontrollable than other variables, has added a new dimension to the study of society.

2. The study of man has made available the means of changing his behaviour if that is so desired. The evolution and refinement of clinical, psychological and sociotherapeutic techniques have enormous implications for the community psychiatric nurse of today and tomorrow, both in terms of patient care and expansion of their role. Indeed, so far has this process gone that Bowart(2) talks about 'psycho-weapons' whilst describing the C.I.A.'s range of psychological warfare techniques.

3. The evolution of behavioural science has fostered the adoption of the 'interdisciplinary approach'. Practitioners, whether from the humanities, the social sciences, the 'natural' sciences or the applied sciences have come together in an effort to pool their knowledge and skills in the attempt to come to terms with the intricacies of human behaviour.

4. It is, perhaps, as a result of all this that we have come to look at human behaviour in a much more enlightened way. We tend to think of it nowadays in terms of not only what people do, i.e. their overt acts—the tip of the iceberg as it were—but also we look at the submerged areas of behaviour: attitudes, expectations, motivations and so forth, all of which eventually dictate the nature of the overt acts which do surface.

The behavioural sciences being a relative newcomer to the academic scene, its boundaries are still quite flexible—the main criterion governing who shall enquire into what, is whether such an exercise will shed any light on a particular aspect of human behaviour.

Its importance for both mental handicap and mental illness nurses working in the community is obvious—behavioural sciences are concerned with precisely that area of knowledge which must constitute the prime focus of the community psychiatric nurse's attention. Community psychiatric nursing needs to grow into the behavioural science traditions of open-mindedness and flexibility. In that way practitioners will see people's problems with more objectivity and will thus avoid the stereotyping that is a hallmark of the institution (cf. Barton(3), Goffman(4)); and they will free themselves from the institutional burden which, as Frost(5) points out, characterises not only the patients but also the staff who work in our psychiatric and mental handicap hospitals.

SECTION A

In this section we shall look at those behavioural sciences which impinge dynamically on the practice of community psychiatric nursing.

As practitioners in what is essentially a new and rapidly expanding field it behoves us to look closely at all the disciplines which can help shed light on our area of practice—and nothing perhaps is more important in this endeavour than the behavioural perspective. As nurses, we are already familiar with the medical perspective—so familiar that it may tend to shut out other 'world views'; we are not, by and large, *au fait* with the behavioural element in nursing practice— certainly not to the extent that is warranted by its importance. This is a sad deficiency in basic training which must inevitably lead to a kind of one-eyed nursing practice—the fault lies not with the nurses themselves but with a system which allows what is manifestly unbalanced and therefore unsuitable training to continue. As far as trained nurses who wish to specialise in a particular area of practice (e.g. child and adolescent psychiatry, behaviour therapy, community psychiatric nursing etc.) are concerned the anomaly can be righted by post-registration training. For the lucky few a more academic diet can be prepared to satisfy their proper needs. But this is only a beginning: not all those who would like to specialise are able, at the moment, to train; and what of those who just want to remain in mainstream mental handicap/psychiatry within an institutional setting? Suffice it at this stage to earnestly entreat all—whatever their preferred field of practice and whether they are able to undertake specialist training or not—to take note of the behavioural perspective in nursing practice. It is applicable in all situations and any care plan which fails to take account of it is only half a care plan, or worse!

Social psychology

Of all the established behavioural sciences, social psychology is perhaps the most crucial in helping community psychiatric nurses to understand the dynamics of human behaviour in the context of mental illness/handicap. This is because amongst other topics social psychology studies 'role', 'social skills' and 'small groups': and these are the very areas of enquiry which are so important in illumining human behaviour.

Role theory

Role theory as such has only been with us since the 1930s. It owes its existence to the writings of many behavioural scientists, but the work of Mead(6), Moreno(7) and Linton(8) have been of paramount importance. 'Role' is also studied by psychology, sociology and anthropology—the emphases and orientations are, of course, quite different in each discipline—and it would not be too great a leap of the imagination to predict that this very important field will draw away from its respective subject area restrictions and will constitute perhaps one of the cornerstones of a behavioural science of the future.

The field, although relatively new, is quite well established—it possesses already a body of knowledge and a language of its own and has developed some theory and characteristic methods of enquiry. The subject matter of role theory is real-life human behaviour as displayed in social situations. Role analysts therefore examine such problems as 'the processes and phases of socialisation, inter-dependence among individuals, the characteristics and organisation of social positions, processes of conformity and functioning, specialisation of performance and the "division of labour"' (Biddle and Thomas(9)). Some concepts developed to explain the nature of the above behaviours include the following:

role category, e.g. mental nurses;

role expectation, i.e. anticipated behaviour associated with a role category;

role behaviour, viz. actions of a person that are relevant to the role he is performing;

role partner, i.e. a person occupying a counterposition to that of the actor, e.g. nurse and patient;

role sectors and role sets: a role set comprises the set of relations which an actor in any social situation has with his role partners, thus for instance a mental handicap nurse's role set will include the relations which the nurse has with patients, social workers, doctors etc.; the role sector will be that set of relationships which exists between any one pair of participants in a role set complex as follows in figure 5.

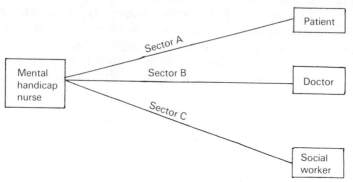

Fig. 5 A role set and some of its role sectors. (After Secord and Backman, *Social Psychology*. New York: McGraw Hill.)

Secord and Backman(10) indicate that normative behaviour i.e. the role expectations associated with any particular role category, have five properties:

1. they shape behaviour in the direction of shared values or desirable states of affairs;
2. they vary in the degree to which they are functionally related to important values;
3. they are enforced by the behaviour of other persons;
4. they vary in how widely they are shared: they may be society-wide or they may belong to small groups;
5. they vary in the range of permissible behaviour.

An actor, e.g. a community psychiatric nurse, cannot play out his role in the work situation without experiencing difficulty from time to time in fulfilling role expectations—the nurse here then is undergoing 'role strain'. If the difficulty encountered is such that it leads to competing or conflicting expectations then the nurse is in a 'role conflict' situation.

It is not too difficult to imagine a situation where nurse, doctor, psychologist and social worker are not in total agreement about how to proceed with regard to a particular patient/client—the nurse's 'role set' in this position then may lead to a 'role strain' or even 'role conflict' situation in respect of one or more 'role sectors'. The reduction of 'role strain' is necessary of course if the fabric of the social situation is not to be rent; the role theorists have consequently explained the various mechanisms and processes whereby this is achieved. Erving Goffman, in *The Presentation of Self in Everyday Life* (11) gives a cynical but amusing account of 'social establishments' where social situations are acted out in such a way as to preserve the system as a relatively closed entity with 'fixed barriers to perception'. Those who have worked in large institutions of any kind e.g. a large psychiatric hospital, will immediately recognise it in the writings of Goffman. The 'community' is also, of course, a 'social establishment' in Goffman's terms, but it is an establishment complicated out of the ordinary by the fact that many other 'social establishments' impinge dynamically upon it. It is essential that all those working in the community—and there is going to be an increasing emphasis on family and the community in the Health and Social Services of the future—it is essential that these practitioners make strenuous efforts to prevent the community from becoming 'closed' and therefore less effective as a therapeutic milieu. One of the ways in which this can be accomplished is through the increased awareness generated by familiarity with the fundamental principles in social psychology, particularly, perhaps, role theory.

Social skills
Probably the most appalling deficiency in mental illness and mental handicap nurse education lies in the area of social skills training. The practice of sending nurses to do their general training has been irrelevant and outmoded for a long time now—if, instead of this, hospitals had sent staff on social skills training courses such as exist in education and industry, we should have made far greater strides in coming to terms with this complex area of human behaviour than indeed is apparent. Having been through the whole process of nurse education/socialisation, the writer believes that general nurse training as it stands is actually detrimental for mental/handicap nurses *vis-à-vis* the acquisition of social skills. One recalls—and many readers will undoubtedly have had similar experiences—being told by a staff nurse; 'come along nurse, you haven't got time to talk to patients here'. Whilst general nursing remains task-orientated then it is no place for the exercise or learning of social skills. The original deliberations of the Briggs Committee (12) concerning psychiatric nursing show how little the members of that committee understood the nature of nurse-patient interaction in the 'distressed person' context. The worst thing that could have happened in terms of the mentally ill in the U.K. would have been for the Briggs Report to have been implemented in its original form.

We have known about social skills training for some years—it is now some ten years since Argyle(13) published his landmark work. We have known about the importance of social skills themselves in psychiatric nursing for much longer—Peplau(14) and Altschul(15) just to mention two have been playing the tune for long enough. The fact that we have made such little progress probably has something to do with the intrinsic nature of this 'fascinating and baffling object of study' (Argyle(13) on 'Social Interaction').

Despite the difficulties inherent in the exercise, the rewards awaiting those who are/become socially competent are immense—to be able to change the behaviour of others has all sorts of exciting implications: the salesman will sell more goods, the foreman will have better relations with his workers, the teacher will be responsible for his students learning more, the football manager will have a more contented playing staff and therefore probably a winning team, the chairman will get through more business in less time and the nurse will be able to help more people more often.

Trower *et al.*(16) characterise the social skills model as follows:

> This model conceptualises man as pursuing social and other goals, acting according to rules monitoring his performance in the light of continuous feedback from the environment.

One of the great breakthroughs in the area of social skills training was made by Argyle(13) in regarding social skills in much the same way as one would look at motor skills. (Motor skills are those involved in the performance of some physical task like playing a particular sport, performing a technical task, etc.) Argyle(13) noted that motor skills had been extensively studied and that their psychological components were well understood, and he went on to suggest that 'social interaction has many resemblances to other motor skills' and that the basic psychological similarities should be looked at in more detail to see if the same processes apply. Processes common to both motor skill and social skill analyses are identified, viz.:

1. the aims of skilled performance;
2. the selective perception of aims;
3. central 'transaction' processes;
4. motor responses;
5. feedback and corrective action; and
6. the timing of responses.

Models are constructed to indicate how these processes apply to both 'motor' and 'social' fields. Argyle(13) then goes on to consider the features which are special to the social skill arena, giving them as follows:

1. the need to establish rapport with the other person;
2. the need to keep the person in play;
3. the need to motivate the client;
4. the need to reduce anxiety, and
5. social performers' concern about the impression they are making on the client.

Is there such a thing as general social competence? In other words, is the person who is a good salesman likely to be a good politician/foreman/chairman/teacher/football manager/disc jockey/therapist?

Argyle(13) thinks this probable:

> ... there is probably some generality about social competence because certain of the elements of skill—for example social sensitivity—are needed in all social situations.

He identifies the components of social competence as follows:

1. perceptual sensitivity;
2. warmth and rapport;
3. repertoire of social techniques;
4. flexibility;
5. energy, and
6. smooth response patterns.

It is clearly of fundamental importance for psychiatric nurses in general to possess and be trained in the use of social skills. (Trower *et al.*(16) state that 'some forms of mental disorder are caused or exacerbated by lack of social competence, and can be cured or alleviated by means of training in social skills'). Yet Altschul(15) as recently as 1972 found that nurses had little conception of 'interpersonal techniques'—considered by Peplau(14) to be the 'crux of psychiatric nursing'. It is of the utmost importance that community psychiatric nurses are well versed in these and other techniques if they are to function even adequately, never mind well. The two skills which are of crucial importance for community psychiatric nurses are:

1. communication skills;
2. interpersonal skills.

On 'the need to establish rapport with other people' Argyle(13) has this to say:

> while everyone has some idea of what is meant by 'rapport', it is by no means clear what it means in terms of interaction sequences. It may be suggested that at least three things are involved. Firstly there must be a clear channel of communication between A and B: they must communicate intelligently so that messages are clearly received.

We need go no further, communication skills are fundamental to any relationship. (Even Skinner(18) has to admit that 'verbal behaviour' is the hallmark of man). Great progress has been made in the field of communications in recent years, as Trower *et al.*(16) note:

> Considerable strides have been made by social psychologists, linguists and sociologists in the study of non-verbal communication, speech and conversation ...

'Communicative competence', as Bell(19) calls it, recognises verbal communication as a social skill as well as a linguistic skill. It is therefore of the utmost importance that those needing to establish rapport—and that must be one of the primary functions of the community psychiatric nurse—understand the nature of communication. Communication has been described as follows:

> ... communication embodies all the modes of behaviour that an individual employs, consciously or unconsciously, to affect another: not only the spoken and written words, but also gestures, body movements, somatic signals and symbolism in the arts. Non-verbal communication as a matter of fact is considered to be a more reliable expression of true feelings than verbal, because the individual has less conscious control over his non-verbal behaviour. Communication functions to mediate information across boundary lines of the human or group organisation, and calls for three necessary operations: perception, evaluation and transmission. 'Perception' is the reception of incoming signals which circulate either inside or outside a human organisation. 'Evaluation' involves summary and analysis of information provided, through retention of past experiences and leads to predictions and decision making. 'Transmission' is expression of information by verbal expression, gestures, movements and social actions. These three basic operations should be looked upon as a unit
>
> (Davis(20)

The acquisition of communication skills is therefore fundamental if the community psychiatric nurse is to act as an agent of behaviour change: 'The core of all psychiatric therapies is the improvements of the communicative behaviour of the patient' (Ruesch21). The same author believes that four characteristics determine whether or not communication is successful:

1. feedback—the mechanism whereby the receiver can relay back to the sender of the message, the effects of the message;
2. appropriateness—the reply is relevant and in keeping with initial statement;
3. efficiency—language simple, messages clear, with enough time for receiver to evaluate;
4. flexibility—neither exaggerated control nor permissiveness.

Any training programme, therefore, which aims to generate/improve communication skills must be based on acquainting the nurse with the various stages of the successful communication process, and then a continual practice until competence is attained. This as Eldred (22) points out, is not simply a question of words but must also involve examination of what gestures, inflections and movements say to people. One way of communicating with a patient/client is via the interview—interviewing is a 'goal directed method of communication—a medium for interaction between two persons' (Greenhill(23). The use of the interview may help to offset what Peplau(14) regards as a possible danger—the use of social chit-chat:

> Talking to patients is easy when the nurse treats the patient as a chum and engages in the give-and-take of social chit-chat. But when the nurse sees her part in verbal exchanges with patients as a major component in direct nursing service, then she must recognise the complexity of the process. Social chit-chat is replaced by the responsible use of words which help to further the personal development of the patient.

Argyle(17) points out how training in social skills can be carried out in a variety of ways:

1. learning on the job: 'The commonest way of learning social skills is through repeated performance in the relevant social situations';
2. role-playing and simulation: 'In role-playing, trainees practise the part they are going to play in a classroom situation, and are given some kind of feedback on their performance';
3. T (training)-groups: '... trainees meet in groups of about 12 for a series of two-hour sessions and their sole task is to study the processes of interaction in the group itself; the leader explains that he is there to help them to do this and occasionally intervenes to comment on what is happening'. Argyle goes on to point out that 'T-group training has far-reaching and comprehensive goals—the overall improvement of social sensitivity, understanding and skill. Here it contrasts with role-playing which is intended to teach specific social skills;'
4. Educational methods of training: lectures and discussions, reading and self-instruction, instructional films.

If communication skills are needed to begin a relationship with a patient, then interpersonal techniques are required to continue that relationship. It is this area that Peplau(14) describes as the 'crux of psychiatric nursing' and it is even more crucial for the community psychiatric nurse than the hospital nurse because there is a greater onus on him/her to seek out the patient and persevere with the relationship. Ideally, interpersonal techniques would consist of a set of strategies for dealing with particular kinds of problem areas e.g. the anxious patient. Once devised by the practitioner these strategies could be put into operation as and when the occasion arose. Carr(24) found that although it was very difficult to get nurses to admit formally to having armouries of strategies the fact that they were so equipped appeared at an informal level. That we should possess such strategies is not surprising since one constantly uses them every day throughout the whole range of interpersonal relationships—what one says and the way one says it to the wife/boss/bank manager will clearly, if one is sensible, vary according to whether they are upset/angry/happy:

> ... if you try to tell them what they do not want to know
> they'll pickle you in piddle
> frizzle you in drizzle
> fry you in the snow

> (Laing 25)

Such strategies can be imparted through a variety of specialised therapies:

1. behaviour therapy;
2. psychotherapy;
3. T-groups;
4. milieu therapy;

but what is really needed for the community psychiatric nurse who (cf. chapter 2) is going to be a 'generalist' is the development of some kind of non-technical psychotherapy. As Orford(26) has noted: 'The word "psychotherapy" is a very general one and covers a multitude of procedures'. Argyle(13) notes '... there is evidence that relatively untrained people can be successful as psychotherapists (Matarozzo, J. D. (1965) Psychotherapeutic processes, *Annual Review of Psychology*, **16**, 181–224); as we have seen, it is the social skill rather than the particular kind of therapy, that counts.' Rogers(27) lists four 'attitudinal patterns' (three in the therapist and one in the patient) which must be present if the relationship is to be successful:

1. 'congruence'—means that the therapist is being himself;
2. 'unconditional positive regard'—means that the therapist experiences an ongoing positive feeling without reservations, without evaluations;
3. 'as if ...'—means that the therapist be experiencing or be as close as possible to experiencing an accurate empathetic understanding;
4. the client/patient must be aware of these attitudes in the therapist—effective communication must have taken place.

What we are really getting at then, is that in this sphere of interpersonal techniques—necessary for the continuance of any meaningful relationship with a patient—the community psychiatric nurse needs to become a good counsellor in order to be successful. 'Being a good counsellor' may be equated with being a 'non-technical psychotherapist'—the title is of little account—possessing/developing the social skills necessary to prolong a relationship until such time as the client finds himself again is what matters. Research is clearly needed in this area of 'counselling strategies for community psychiatric nurses', and one could do much worse than to start off at the point where Trower *et al.*(16) finished in their recent work. In their training manual they list ten main areas of social deficiency, and discuss the following skills:

> observation skills;
> listening skills;
> speaking skills;
> meshing skills;
> expression of attitudes;
> social routines;
> tactics and strategies;
> situation training.

Any one of these areas could be researched from the viewpoint of community psychiatric nursing, and the knowledge gained could not but help those working in the community to become more effective practitioners.

Small groups

Much of what has been said so far in this chapter comes together in the group situation. Hollander(28) observes: 'Groups carry out their operations within a structure'. Three features of structure are the 'status differentiation' within the group, its 'norms', and its 'communication pattern'. Norms and status are interrelated in so far as specialised roles are created for a person occupying a given status. In this sense a role can be thought of as a highly specialised norm within the role system which characterises any group. The nature of structure affects 'interaction' within groups. Hollander(28) further notes that groups may be looked at from two standpoints:

1. the group level—where one is interested in 'performance'— somtimes called 'task groups' e.g. the levels of cohesiveness, solidarity, communication and conformity; and
2. the individual level—where one is interested in members' satisfaction—sometimes called 'growth groups', e.g. levels of

motivation and affiliation as represented by such concepts as 'social identity', 'social reality' and 'social support'.

Taylor and Kleinhans(29) define a group as follows: 'a collection of two or more persons who interact in the context of shared norms and goals'. The heading of this section is 'small groups'—how big is small? Taylor and Kleinhans(29) proffer Bales(30) suggestion in relation to the size of a small group:

> Each member receives some impression or perception of each other member enough so that he can either at the time or in later questioning, give some reaction to each of the others as an individual person even though it be only to recall that the other person was present

(Bales R. F. (1950) *Interaction Process Analysis: A method for the study of small groups*. Reading, Mass.: Addison-Wesley,(30)). Groups of fewer than 20 are thought by many to be right for a 'small group'; and clearly size is very important in relation to the small group. Steiner(31) remarks (per Taylor and Kleinhans): 'for most tasks groups productivity increases with group size up to a certain point, after which it levels off and then declines.' A large task group has certain advantages over a small group. Large groups generally have greater member resources. On the other hand large groups have difficulties in the areas of organisation and motivation. Beyond a certain size, the disadvantages outweigh the advantages and group performance declines. When it comes to the 'growth group', viz. the kind of group concerned with the satisfaction of the individual members of the group, then the optimum size is quite small. Kleinhans and Taylor(32) note:

> Slater[33], measured the satisfaction of members of discussion groups varying in size from two to seven. The members of five-person groups expressed the greatest satisfaction with their group size. Dissatisfaction with larger groups centred on organisational problems and lack of opportunity to participate. The members of smaller groups may have felt they lacked a sufficiently wide range of viewpoints to analyse the discussion topic satisfactorily.

Whether one belongs to a particular group or not is unimportant at the social-psychological level—what matters is that the importance of group activity is recognised in human behaviour. Argyle(17) observes

> A great deal of social interaction takes place in small social groups. Monkeys and apes live in groups, within which children are procreated and reared with various family structures. The work of gathering food and drink and arranging shelter is performed, leisurely social activities occur and defence against predators is organised. This is presumably an instinctive pattern of behaviour, which has evolved through the survival of those groups and their members that adopted it. Human life is similar: children are reared in families, go out to play with groups of friends, are educated in groups at school; later they work in co-operative groups and live in families of their own, which form communities and they pursue common interests in various societies and clubs.

The three most important groups according to Argyle(17) are:

1. the family;
2. work-groups, and
3. groups of friends.

A very interesting account of 'interaction' within these three groups is given by Argyle(17) but it is no part of our task to elaborate on this here.

What does need further comment at this point is another kind of group activity, invented by psychologists, viz. T-groups and therapy groups. The former group consists of a number of trainees—usually between 10 and 15—and a trainer, and they meet for a specific period of time to study the group; the latter group, however, usually consists of a smallish group of mental patients, often less than 10, and a therapist, and the basic function is to make use of the group's behaviour in diagnosing basic personality disturbances. This type of activity—in which the members are concerned with their own experiences—is the sort of activity which is important in the context of community psychiatric nursing. Here groups are not concerned with an extrinsic goal and the role of the group leader—of great importance in groups so concerned—is rather muted and quite distinctive. The leader is a sort of anachronistic figure in that the role had become formalised around informal behaviour. The T-group can be utilised to train the would-be therapist and the therapy group is a very suitable medium for the community psychiatric nurse to interact with certain groups of patients in order to try and bring about a change in disturbed behaviour, and even, if possible, effect long-term changes in attitude and behaviour. As Gahagan(34) notes: the growth of 'personal relationship groups' as opposed to 'groups with extrinsic goals' represents an important step forward in psychology; it would be a great opportunity lost were community psychiatric nurses and psychiatric nurses generally to fail in seizing hold of the chances offered by these techniques to improve patient care and extend the roles of nurse practitioners.

Groups, of course, afford the opportunity to all participants to practise social skills through role play: for patients, skills which are important in ordinary everyday life; for professionals, skills which they will need over and over again in their jobs. Klein(35) observes: 'Role playing gives an opportunity to practise roles which are required in these situations but which tend to be performed inadequately because they are not naturally congenial.' Argyle(13) remarks: 'The main effect of role-playing, however, is probably to accelerate the acquisition of skill in the performance of social techniques'. Community psychiatric nurses must develop social competence if they are to become well-rounded practitioners (generalists rather than narrow specialists), and the small group is at one and the same time a learning context and a therapeutic medium.

Social psychiatry

A s a term social psychiatry can be used in a general sense—to denote the broad range of pyschiatric practice today, and in a specialist sense—to describe the scope of the social model in mental illness. As a field of enquiry it embraces elements of both the medical and the behavioural sciences. Its importance for community psychiatric nurses is seminal in that community mental health is the province of a number of different kinds of practitioners, often operating with differing philosophical orientations. (The possible combinations of personnel and philosophy are described by Siegler and Osmond(36) as follows:

1. Doctors using a medical model.
2. Doctors using a non-medical model.
3 Non-medical personnel using a medical model.
4. Non-medical personnel using a non-medical model.).

It will not, therefore, be possible for community psychiatric nurses to operate effectively unless the main strands of thought and practice running through social psychiatry are understood.

The fundamentalist ideas underlying the practice of social psychiatry have already been sketched out in brief in Chapter 2. Perhaps the major triumph to date of social psychiatry has been the development of these basic philosophical notions into a coherent system of ideological orientations known as models of mental illness. When the medical model as we know it was 'king', discussion of models for dealing with mental illness was unheard of and indeed not necessary, since the existence of alternatives was not perceived. The arrival of alternatives, opening up new sets of possibilities, has lead to a debate which has had a fundamental bearing on thinking and practice in psychiatry and which has great implications for the development of community psychiatric nursing. As Siegler and Osmond(36) point out: 'They [the models] have allowed an ordering of well known facts and inquiry into other facts which were less known or hardly known at all, which would not have otherwise been understood simply because there would have been no particular reason to do so'. For instance, consider the word 'cure' and listen to what David Cooper(37) has to say about it;

> Curing is so ambiguous a term; one may cure bacon, hides, rubber, or patients. Curing usually implies the chemical treatment of raw materials so that they may taste better, be more useful, or last longer. Curing is technically a mechanistic perversion of medical ideals that is quite opposite in many ways to the authentic tradition of healing.

Sentiments such as these could clearly never have been uttered prior to the evolution of social psychiatry.

It would be premature to claim that a satisfactory body of knowledge exists but, as Orford(26) has noted: 'The idea that behaviour can be interpreted in various different ways, or that different constructions can be placed upon other people's behaviour, provides a major theme'. This theme now has a considerable number of theoretical variations and these have been characterised by a goodly number of writers within the last decade. The resulting miasma of models and sub-models has been brought together in a masterly analysis and exposition by Siegler and Osmond(36) on whom the following resume relies:

1. *Discontinuous models*—models that put forth a partial or restricted view of the problem of madness:

a. The Medical Model

tends to view things in terms of:

   (i) the patient;

   (ii) the hospital;

   (iii) an examination;

   (iv) the diagnosis;

   (v) treatment;

   (vi) prognosis.

b. The Moral Model

tends to look at the 'patient' as 'bad' rather than 'mad'. Disgusting or unusual behaviour provokes an interpretation of the 'patient' which takes the form of labelling, i.e. deviant behaviour. Interestingly, as Orford(26) observes, the act of labelling is itself a form of deviance 'a form of secondary deviance which may be more harmful than the primary deviancy to which it was a reaction'. Those who set out to correct abnormal behaviour and bring it within acceptable limits (usually without too much concern for its origin) may be said to be choosing a moral model of madness. (Behaviour therapy/modification set out to correct abnormal behaviour of course!)

c. The Impaired Model

tends to see the 'patient' as impaired. Treatment is not important unless a scientific advance makes impairment a treatable condition. Rehabilitation is the watchword, and the degree of impairment will be crucial in determining what can be achieved. The worst factor of caring for the impaired in institutions is that no change is expected for either better or worse.

2. *Continuous models*—models that seek a total explanation of madness:

a. The Psychoanalytic Model

tends to look upon the disturbed person not as suffering from a disease but as a victim of some grievous error of child-rearing. (Psychotherapy of course seeks to redress such errors!)

b. The Social Model

tends to view society as the cause of disturbed behaviour in people. Change—especially rapid change (cf. Toffler(38))—is seen as pathological. Some radical social psychiatrists even go so far as to say that the only way to eliminate mental illness is to revolutionise society. (Sociotherapy uses the group/community as a therapeutic medium for the group/community).

c. The Psychedelic Model

tends to view madness as a mind-expanding trip and suggests that those who make the journey will somehow see things more clearly. R. D. Laing(25) is the arch-exponent of this view today.

d. The Conspiratorial Model

asks the very pertinent question 'does madness exist at all?' May it not only be present—like beauty—in the eye of the beholder? This model owes much to the writings of Szasz(39) and Goffman(11) and is the one most often associated with the term 'antipsychiatry'.

e. The Family Interaction Model

tends to view the family as the fundamental unit of conceptualisation with the implication that troubled families make member(s) ill. (Family therapy is naturally the therapy of choice!)

We have alluded *en passant* to:

> behaviour therapy/modification;
> psychotherapy; and
> sociotherapy.

It is now time to say a little more about these regimes and their importance for the community psychiatric nurse.

1. Behaviour therapy (behaviour modification)

As has been mentioned in Chapter 2, behaviour therapy is a product of 'behaviourism' founded by Watson(40) who in turn owed much to the ideas of Pavlov(41). As such the term 'behaviour therapy' was coined in

1954 by Skinner and Lindsley(42). Eysenck(43) is perhaps the key figure in the field today and has played a very influential part in behaviour therapy gaining the wide acceptance which it currently enjoys.

Many definitions of the regime exist:

> The behaviouristic approach . . . has been characterised by the attempt to apply laboratory methods and controls to the study and modification of abnormal forms of behaviour
>
> Yates(44)

> Behaviour therapy . . . is the use of experimentally-established principles of learning for the purpose of changing unadaptive behaviour. Unadapted habits are weakened and eliminated: adaptive habits are initiated and strengthened.
>
> Wolpe(45)

Underlying the practice of such a regime is the philosophical notion—sinister if taken to the ultimate extreme—that man is a mechanism; that as a mechanism he can be controlled if we know enough about him/it. The pervasive logic of the proposition is positively Orwellian(46) in its implications.

On the other hand nobody can doubt that behaviour therapy/modification techniques can be, and are, extremely useful. We have come a long way from the 'habit training wards' of yesteryear as Wolpe(45) notes:

> Before the advent of behaviour therapy, psychological medicine was a medley of speculative systems and intuitive methods. Behaviour therapy is an applied science, in every way parallel to other modern technologies and in particular those that constitute modern medical therapeutics.

We shall now look very briefly at the main technologies which go to make up the field:

a. Systematic desensitisation.

Yates(44) describes it as follows:

> a general set of experimental procedures that may involve the use of either or both of the procedures defined as counter conditioning (reciprocal inhibition) and extinction. Its use, according to Wolpe(45) is that it 'is one of a variety of methods for breaking down neurotic anxiety-response habits in piecemeal fashion, modelled on the therapy of experimental neurosis. A psychological state inhibitory of anxiety is induced in the patient by means of muscle relaxation and he is then exposed to a weak anxiety-arousing stimulus for a few seconds. If the exposure is repeated several times, the stimulus progressively loses its ability to evoke anxiety. Then successively 'stronger' stimuli are introduced and similarly treated

There are quite a number of variations of systematic desensitisation, e.g. group desensitisation and automated desensitisation involving the use of relaxation tapes.

b. Procedure provoking strong anxiety.

In systematic desensitisation it is usual for a gradual progression to be made through a hierarchy from the least to the most anxiety-provoking event (stimulus). Here, however, that is not the case—the patient is as it were, thrown in at the deep end in an effort to rid him of his phobia. A number of techniques are based on this formula:

(i) flooding—
the subject is exposed *in vivo* to the most anxiety provoking stimulus and from which escape is impossible;

(ii) implosive theory—
the subject is exposed, imaginally, to the stimulus which he fears and from which he cannot escape;

(iii) abreaction—
memories of distressful events are stirred up in the subject in order to evoke a strong response.

c. Operant-conditioning procedures.
Techniques used in this area rely in general on the experimental work of Skinner(18) and his associates (cf. Wolpe(45)). The techniques are as follows:

(i) positive reinforcement—
basically a reward of some kind or other, e.g. food, money etc.;

(ii) negative reinforcement—
removal of undesirable stimulus after appropriate response;

(iii) extinction—
progressive weakening of a response by the removal of reinforcement in the face of the continuing response;

(iv) differential reinforcement—
a selective combination of positive reinforcement and extinction;

(v) shaping—
a special example of positive reinforcement;

(vi) punishment—
an aversive stimulus is given to the subject following the undesirable response.

These techniques are used most widely in the treatment of childhood psychoses and behaviour problems in adult psychoses, in the care of those who exhibit anti-social tendencies, and of course in mental handicap.

d. Aversion Therapy.
This consists in administering an aversive stimulus in order to prevent an undesired response, in the hope that the strength of the habit will be diminished. Aversive stimuli may be applied in a

number of ways:
(i) electric shock—
usually administered to a limb;
(ii) drugs—
well known in the treatment of alcoholism;
(iii) paralysis—
for instance, in the treatment of alcoholism;
(iv) covert sensitisation—
the pairing of a verbally suggested aversive response with an imagined stimulus;
(v) intense illumination and white noise—
these techniques have been used and call to mind how close to 'third degree treatment' aversion therapy may come;
(vi) other aversive agents—
consisting of anything that is unpleasant—like foul-smelling liquids or gases, shame etc.

The use of aversion therapy lies mainly in the area of obsessive-compulsive behaviour, fetishism, homosexuality, alcoholism, smoking, drug-addiction. This is clearly only intended to be a brief outline of the field in order to point out its relevance for the community psychiatric nurse. The range of disorders treatable by behaviour therapy/modification is large and includes many of the problem areas which the community psychiatric nurse—mental handicap or mental illness practitioner—daily comes into contact with. A knowledge of the field is necessary if for nothing more than to recognise the potential which exists for helping people with a particular form of disturbed behaviour. In order to bring home to the reader the importance of this field for the community psychiatric nurses we are giving the following care-study to illustrate the point.

Behaviour therapy care study

Operant conditioning. This, in essence, is rewarding behaviour as it occurs. The importance of operant behaviour is that it can be reinforced, increasing the likelihood of its recurrence resulting in some change in behaviour, or learning to have taken place without being aware of the motivation, cause, drive or stimulus of that behaviour.

By selectively reinforcing behaviour deemed to be desirable, a person's performance may be modified to conform with target behaviour selected by the operator. The power should also generate responsibility. Certainly many instances of unkindness, malpractice even ill-treatment have arisen as a direct result of the use, or rather mis-use, of the techniques of behaviour modification. The monitoring of any behavioural techniques used in the home needs to be considered. Regular review of programmes, methods and progress should be undertaken by the community team.

In order to establish a desired behaviour the target behaviour must be potentially available. Any behaviour that approximates to the desired behaviour must be rewarded. This is termed 'shaping'. The reward must immediately follow the response. The reward for reinforcer can only be so described if the chances of the behaviour recurring are increased. The person must be known to respond to reinforcement, and the effective reinforcement, be it social approval, a Smartie, Twiglet or the opportunity for some self indulgence, (watching television or going for a walk). The desired response must only be rewarded if competing or unwanted behaviours are absent so that undesirable responses are not rewarded and thus not reinforced.

Although we are not aware of cues that initiate or affect behaviour it is possible to establish some degree of cue control. If particular places are used for particular activities, then features of the environment will affect the behaviour. Two contrasting aspects of mental retardation concern the response to cues. On the one hand the inability to discriminate results in the person making general, behaviour that should be specific, e.g. urinating everywhere. Failure to generalise results from too rigid cues, e.g. only using one toilet; some effort needs to be made to establish cue control, avoiding rigidity.

Prompting may be physical, verbal or mixed. It is a discriminatory stimulus encouraging correct response. This may take the form of a direct command, go to the toilet, or be supplemented by a gesture, e.g. pointing to the toilet. Much of normal social behaviour is learned by prompting. When used as part of a programme of training it is important that the same prompt is given on each occasion and not to say toilet on one occasion and lavatory or loo on another.

Fading (or the case of the diminishing cue) occurs when the degree of prompting is progressively reduced, by reducing the number of words, giving the first part of the word, or lowering the voice when a verbal prompt is given. The principle is the same with non-verbal physical cues.

A simple example illustrates how errors can occur if a programme is improperly monitored or executed. A person was being instructed in the use of the 'Green Cross Code' to cross a road. The prompt of 'road drill' evoked the appropriate road crossing behaviour. When subsequently approaching a kerb-side no 'Green Cross' appeared the person stepped directly out into the road. The cue for appropriate road crossing behaviour was not a road kerb but someone saying 'road drill' in the left ear. Had the prompt been faded correctly, the kerb would have become established as the cue for 'Green Cross' behaviour. To extend the illustration—this behaviour must become generalised, as a too rigid cue control would result in the behaviour not being evoked at a position where it may be more important.

Following 'reinforcement', 'shaping', 'prompting' and 'fading'; to complete this small compass of behavioural aspects of teaching the mentally retarded mention must be made of 'extinction'. If behaviour occurs, something somewhere must be reinforcing it. Extinction, or cessation of the response occurs when it is no longer rewarded or rewards are given for incompatible behaviours; i.e. rewarding standing to eliminate sitting.

When establishing any programme it is important to be aware of current undesirable behaviour being reinforced and in what manner. We tend to assume that children arrive with a 'hand-book' on how they should be reared, consequently parents reinforce behaviour which may not be appropriate, rewarding attention—seeking behaviour whatever form that takes. The elimination of some desirable behaviour may result from its not being rewarded.

It is not proposed here to give any details about reinforcement schedules or the many refinements of the techniques involved in behaviour modification. Research has shown that, although reading and discussion can impart knowledge and change attitudes, the effect on behaviour is minimal. The only effective way of learning about behaviour modification is to undertake a programme with expert guidance. Community nurses should avail themselves of the opportunity of undergoing training in this most useful of techniques, thereby not only knowing the methods but also the limitations.

The intended use of a behavioural modification programme and its implementation demands a similar pattern as is described elsewhere, namely the nursing process: Assessment-Objective-Content-Method-Re-assessment-Evaluation.

The initial assessment provides a base-line of performance against which subsequent behavioural changes can be measured. Objective— a measurable behavioural change—the target behaviour. How is the change to be brought about? Extinction, cue control, selective reinforcement (on what schedule), forward or reverse chaining, type and degree of prompt? How are records to be maintained, by whom? What date is fixed for the re-assessment?

Consider the problem of an incontinent child at home. A base-line of incontinence must be established by accurate observation and recording over a two-week period. Does he indicate he wishes to go to the toilet, does he go if prompted or does he need to be taken. Does he unfasten his trousers, needing prompting or help. Similarly with taking his trousers/underpants down. Does he sit down, require prompting or to be gently restrained; does urination/defaecation take place?

Having established a base-line of behaviour properly recorded a programme to reduce the incidence of incontinence must then be implemented. How often is toileting to take place and how long each session, at what time in relation to his established pattern? Starting with the times he has previously been incontinent gradually increasing the sessions from three to four up to eight or ten per day of ten minutes each.

The profile of current behaviour must be compared with target behaviour i.e. going to the toilet, eliminating appropriately, undressing, dressing—independently of direction. The toileting behaviour may thus involve complex sub-divisions of the task so that small gradations can be reinforced thereby 'shaping' the behaviour. This involves rewarding appropriate toileting behaviour immediately it occurs. Inappropriate toileting behaviour, including incontinence should be ignored. Being unaware of the cue it is possible to reinforce unwanted behaviour by the giving of attention. Nurses find it difficult to change a patient without showing disapproval or giving attention; do not think parents will find it any easier!

With this schedule of reinforcement and frequent toileting the incontinence should diminish. The next step is to 'fade the prompt' for each stage and to generalise the behaviour to other toilets.

After a period of six to eight weeks a new base-line must be established and the programme examined to evaluate to what extent the objective of continence had been reached and to identify further training areas.

For the child who plays with food he should be removed from table and 'no' said firmly to him. Removing him prevents further reward being obtained from his activity. He should be returned to the table when he is not exhibiting moulding behaviour. By not using the same table for play-dough, plasticine or clay modelling, cue control should be established assisting the child to discriminate between when moulding activity is appropriate and when it is not.

Needless to say all programmes should be properly set up and properly monitored, and the ethics of modifying behaviour borne in mind.

The difference between everyday life and behaviour modification is that in the former, reinforcement is casual and erratic, whereas in the latter it is systematised, programmed and consistently applied. In life each is modifying the behaviour of the other, without necessarily always being aware. Operant conditioning can seem 'clinical' and dehumanising, and in its extreme form may be so in the short term, but it gives a 'ticket' to a fuller life.

Understanding the basic principles can make life more enjoyable for many, including parents of the handicapped if they can be shown how *not* to reinforce undesirable behaviour.

2. *Psychotherapy*

In contrast to behaviour therapy which is more or less a twentieth-century phenomenon, psychotherapy can be traced in one form or another right back to ancient societies. As Kreeger(47) notes:

> there is evidence that the Shamans of certain Siberian tribes practised hypnotism. Primitive disease theories include such concepts as loss of the soul, sorcery, breech of taboo and spirit intrusion. As a result of very simple cause and effect reasoning, therapy included the finding and restoration of the soul, counter-magic, confession and propitiation and exorcism ...
>
> The Greeks, whilst taking a basically philosophical view of disease, were very much aware of psychological disturbances ...
>
> The Hindu culture also developed an elaborate medical system in which mental disorders remained largely the domain of priestly metaphysics.

Psychotherapy as we know it today however, may be said to have begun with Freud(48) at the beginning of the twentieth century, and is based on the so-called 'psychoanalytical model of mental illness'. Freud broke from the tradition of Mesmer, Braid and Charcot involving the use of hypnotic techniques and founded the psychoanalytic movement. He sought, through self-analysis and analysis of others, to construct a body of theory concerning the structure of the mind and you will all be familiar with his concepts of the id, the ego and the super-ego as the combatants of the unconscious.

The psychoanalytic movement attracted many able people who in turn left their respective marks in distinctive ways:

Carl Jung, who founded the school of analytical psychology;

Alfred Adler, who founded the school of individual psychology;

Anna Freud—Freud's daughter—who contributed much to child analysis;

Melanie Klein who was also very active in the field of child analysis;

Adolf Meyer who pioneered the psychoanalytical approach;

Carl Rogers(27) who involved himself in client-centred therapy;

Eric Berne who originated transactional analysis—an exciting way of looking at manipulative communication—particularly in the family context;

J. C. Moreno who concentrated his efforts in the area of psychodrama; and

the existentialist school focussing on the reality of existence, prominent amongst whom are Ronald Laing(25) and David Cooper(37).

Psychotherapy can be viewed as a number of schools—each with its own particular orientation: Freudian, Jungian, Kleinian, Adlerian—and each with its own dedicated devotees. It is no part of our task to explore the current balance and status of the respective schools—for that the reader must turn to the texts specifically written to that end, q.v. the bibliography at the end of this chapter; rather we are at pains (as we are throughout the whole of this chapter) to point out the relevance of a particular field of knowledge to the community psychiatric nurse. The relevance in the case of psychotherapy is clearly manifold and pervasive:

1. Family Therapy—'Family Therapy can be defined as the psychotherapeutic treatment of a natural social system' (Wolrand-Skinner(49)).

2. Marital Therapy—'Marital Therapy is a form of psychotherapy in that a trained person establishes a professional contract with the patient-couple and through definite types of communication, attempts to alleviate the disturbance, reverse or change maladaptive patterns of behaviour and encourage personality growth and development' (Freedman, Kaplan and Sadock(50)).

3. Group Therapy—a good example of which would be the T-group, where individuals come together as a sensitivity group of one kind or another.

Whilst group psychotherapy has undoubtedly expanded significantly in recent years it must be said that individual psychotherapy remains the cornerstone of the method. The application of this technique is of course determined by the needs of the client—whether child, adolescent or adult—and individual psychotherapy is practised both under the National Health Service and privately.

Psychotherapy is, therefore, clearly significant for community psychiatric nurses whether on an individual counselling basis or in a group-supportive context. In the future, its importance must increase in relation to the practice of community psychiatric nursing. The community psychiatric nurse is a 'generalist', i.e. one who is able when confronted by illness behaviour to review the totality of treatment possibilities and select according to the needs of the particular patient/client. Psychotherapy is an essential element in the treatment spectrum, whether on its own or used in combined treatment. The advent of the crisis-intervention team and the likely continued increase in the use of the same is bringing closer the day when the community psychiatric nurse may be called upon to offer instant counselling to severely disturbed people. While this places a heavy burden on the community psychiatric nurse it is a burden that should not be shirked since it calls to mind the foremost goal of community psychiatric nursing—primary prevention.

Psychotherapy care study

Introduction. Psychotherapy has its 'gurus' and devotees who have worked long and hard in the search for 'the definitve therapy'. The fact of a shift in emphasis from institution to community will not radically alter the sympathisers or antagonists of psychotherapy. As is argued elsewhere, the move from hospital to community does not require a complete new person/professional; it requires more of a shift in emphasis. From Freud to Rogers has seen a number of changes in approach to psychotherapy and the community psychiatric nurse will really have to decide which methods he wishes to use and to what extent he wishes to use them. Some methods lend themselves more easily to the 'community' than do others and some samples will be shown here.

It is worth initially looking at the therapist. If that is what the community psychiatric nurse wishes to be we will assume that as a registered nurse he will have gained some experience as a therapist or group leader in the ward, day hospital or out-patient setting. It is not however the place of this book to indicate training methods and minimum experience time for practising psychotherapists. Psychotherapy in its most rudimentary form (supportive psychotherapy) is a vital constituent part of the community psychiatric nurse's overall role and those not wishing to utilise this part of their work will miss out in large areas of care. It is, therefore, more important to differentiate between supportive psychotherapy and interpretive psychotherapy.

Supportive psychotherapy. Supportive psychotherapy is an important feature of the community psychiatric nurse's role. It is possible to identify constituent parts of the dynamics of supportive psychotherapy.

The therapist will have a good history and knowledge of the patient which should enable him to assess without bias or criticism the stress-provoking factors in the overall picture presented by the patient. The role of the therapist is partially one of a ventilator/leaning post which patients can use when they feel the need to express their feelings and problems. The patient may well invite the community psychiatric nurse to comment or criticise on the information given. The community psychiatric nurse should preferably offer openings to the patient along which they can move themselves and attain a fuller self-realisation.

One of the vital factors is, of course, time. Where many professionals have not got the time to sit down and talk to people and consequently gain their confidence and trust, the community psychiatric nurse is ideally suited to this purpose.

The initial moves to community psychiatric nursing can often result in the community psychiatric nurse receiving those patients with whom other people have tried and failed, and supportive psychotherapy with the community psychiatric nurse is seen as the last resort. Quite often the reason for these failures is that previous supportive psychotherapy is ill-conceived and not carried out with any thought. The following points are worth bearing in mind when considering supportive psychotherapy:

1. Time
Time must be allocated for the session to take place and five minutes pushed in here and there is of very limited value.

2. Relationship formation
Some form of relationship must develop before supportive psychotherapy can take place. A trusting relationship can only develop if the 'therapist' is reliable and turns up when promised and gives the allocated time as arranged.

3. Content
The extent and limitations of the relationship should be discussed and the 'helping' rather than the 'curative' aspects of the relationship should be noted. A patient's expectations of supportive psychotherapy may well differ from those of the community psychiatric nurse. The patient may well consider it important to go off into the areas of self-analysis, something the community psychiatric nurse may not be able to cope with and so any such problems should be sorted out as soon as possible.

Case study of supportive psychotherapy
Mrs S was referred to the community psychiatric nurse by her general practitioner as he was unsure how to manage this particular case. Mrs S was 63 years of age and her husband who was two years older than her was in the fourth year of a long-standing depressive illness. He had been admitted to hospital on a number of occasions after threatening suicide and showing violent outbursts directed towards his wife. Mr S was diagnosed as an arteriosclerotic dementia on his last admission to hospital and only his wife had been told. He was unaware of this diagnosis and was kept in ignorance after a joint decision between Mrs S and the consultant. Prior to his illness Mr and Mrs S had run a ladies' and gents' hairdressing shop. The shop was modest but paid its way and all the business details were taken care of by Mr S. One year ago he lost all interest in the shop. Mrs S was now visiting her General Practitioner regularly and complaining of anxiety and depression.

The community psychiatric nurse visited Mrs S and found out the following relevant information. Mr and Mrs S had no family and kept themselves to themselves very much. On interview Mrs S said she could not talk to anyone about the way she felt as it was too personal and very complicated. The community psychiatric nurse set out a regular appointment when he called to see Mrs S and offered her 7×1 hour sessions. The following problems had been aired and talked through:

1. Mrs S was unused to business affairs and the business was suffering as a consequence; this was talked through and Mrs S enlisted professional accounting help;

2. Mrs S was obviously concerning about the fact of hiding her husband's diagnosis from him. This fact was talked through and she reached a firm decision to keep this to herself but was now convinced she had valid reasons for doing so;

3. Mrs S was very concerned about the future; with the community psychiatric nurse's professional advice, contingency plans were decided.

Comments. Without taking a direct part in the decision making of Mrs S the community psychiatric nurse helped her arrive at a number of decisions of her own free will. The community psychiatric nurse acted purely as a catalyst in this setting, supporting and advising where necessary. Mrs S was obviously in need of such a helping facility as she was trapped in a circle of difficult decisions and her inability to talk them through with anyone and subsequently arrive at a decision was provoking anxiety and depression. The 'support' and 'talk' elements are vital to supportive psychotherapy.

Interpretive psychotherapy. This specialist area includes such therapies as psychoanalysis, analytical psychology, individual psychology, group psychotherapy and transactional analysis.

These different therapies all vary in their approaches to psychotherapy and they will not be detailed here. Psychiatric nurses in particular have been subjected to the fancies and vagaries of each new 'revolutionary therapy' as it has come along and this has not unnaturally left a healthy suspicion of some of the psychotherapy schools. It is as well to say that unless the community psychiatric nurse is prepared to undergo a thorough training in one or other of the various schools of thought connected with psychotherapy it is best not to dabble half-heartedly in these areas. A poorly-defined or amateurish analysis is worse than none at all.

3. Sociotherapy

The 'social model of mental illness' on which the sociotherapeutic approach is based is of quite recent origin. It owes its existence to the writings (mostly in the late fifties and early sixties) of a very influential group which includes such people as:

Maxwell Jones(51)
Thomas Szasz(39)
Marie Jahoda(52)
Thomas Scheff(53)
Erving Goffman(11) and
Howard Becker(54)

The very term 'social psychiatry' if used in the specialist sense, is descriptive of the social model and its concomitant 'milieu therapy' orientation and calls to mind primarily the writers mentioned above.

Underlying the 'social model of mental illness' is the whole area of deviance and social control. This area, of such importance in sociology and social psychiatry, has been a fruitful source of theory for writers in the field of mental health. Concepts such as:

socialisation;
symbolic interaction;
stereotyping;
scape-goating;
stigma,

spring readily to mind when discussion of the 'social model' arises.

The 'social model of mental illness' is based on the assumption that mental illness arises out of society itself, by virtue of its structure and functions. Many writers—in particular psychiatrists who, of course being doctors, have been socialised to consider illness behaviour as an illness phenomenon and the person exhibiting it as an individual patient—make the fundamental mistake when putting forth their views on the 'social model' of treating it in relation to the individual patient. If one is dealing with a social model then one must analyse in terms of a social paradigm i.e one which looks on the patient/client/ sufferer/sinner/deviant *not* as an individual—to do so would be to adopt a psychologistic stance—but as one who occupies a certain position in society. What a particular position entails for any individual who occupies it can only be appreciated if the mechanisms of society are understood. If on mature reflection the mechanisms of society are seen to be in some way faulty, then as sure as night follows day the units that go to make up such a society will similarly in some way also be faulty. Goffman(11), Scheff(53) and Becker(54) in particular have shown up faulty structures in society and have characterised the processes which occur whereby units (individuals occupying certain positions in society) are punished/labelled/stigma-tised in order that the social control mechanism may be brought to bear to preserve the *raison d'être* of that society. The label therefore, 'mental illness', tells one as much about a society as it does about a particular individual living within that society: conferment of the label represents nothing more than a value-judgement even when it comes from the best qualified and most enlightened of social control agents.

If 'illness' is experienced by any one member of a community then—to adopt the sociotherapeutic approach—that community must be accorded the 'sick role' and a therapy programme based on the consensus of the group planned and implemented. The scope of the programme will clearly depend on a variety of factors—age, sex, whether the person is an in-patient or an out-patient, whether the person is in employment or not, the family profile, the resources of the health and social agencies—to name but a few. There can be little doubt that there is a big role for the community psychiatric nurse in this field since it is the community or society, large or small, that one is undertaking to care for. Of the four key members in this area: doctor, nurse, psychologist, social worker, it is the nurse only who is fully equipped to deal with the wide spectrum of behaviour. Others may be strong in certain areas—the doctor in pathology, the psychologist in clinical features, the social worker in some social aspects—the community psychiatric nurse being a generalist, is versed in all these areas and as such is the person most likely to be able to deliver a balanced care programme to the group/community.

The form the group therapy will take will obviously depend on the factors involved. The mechanics may differ little in fact from group psychotherapy but the emphasis will be quite different. Whereas in group psychotherapy the group is used to help the individual, in sociotherapy the collective units of a group are brought together for the group's own good. If the group can be 'cured' then the behaviour of the individuals composing that group will no longer be abnormal. Fears are often expressed (cf. Clare(55)) as to the size of the treatment group and thus the competence of the therapist. (Clare, incidentally, seems to consider this a problem only for the psychiatrist whom he sees as a sort of superivsory social engineer spreading himself ever more thinly towards the boundaries of society's unhappiness!) The problem is naturally one for all the professionals involved. The community psychiatric nurse, while taking account of the fact that a community may be sick—high unemployment for instance—will need also to bear in mind the logistics of any large-scale operation. As in all referral situations, careful screening is a 'must'; much will depend on current case-loads commitments, ratio per 1000 population, teamwork resources and back-up facilities.

It remains nevertheless a challenge to community psychiatric nursing—and indeed to the whole of the nursing profession—that it should begin to think more of community care in the full sense of the term. If the ideal of prevention is ever to be achieved in any field it must be done out there in society and not in the institutions.

Sociotherapy care study

Introduction. Sociotherapy, if applied in its widest context, has much to offer to the community psychiatric nurse. The idea of the 'social self' raises the question of how to make available a means of looking at oneself in a social setting and how to take account of and use the 'deviances' displayed by people to modify isolating behaviour or to produce a normalising effect.

Sociotherapy is the basic move from institution to social care. The placing of care and treatment in a community rather than a hospital setting is one of the fundamental principles of community psychiatric nursing. One major problem which faces the community psychiatric nurse is the possibility that he may carry the principles of the institution with him into the community. It is a feature of 'the community' that it will not tolerate the ways of institutional care as they are likely to show up as 'odd' or 'strange' when seen in the community.

One method which uses sociotherapy heavily is the social group or club. Where such groups exist they cater for different types of clientele ranging from

a. the active socialising group which consciously trys to re-socialise the isolated.

to

b. groups which meet purely as means of coming together for tea and company. It will depend very much on the aims of such a group as to the way it is run.

A deliberate attempt by staff can be made to use such a group for a specific purpose. The tea-and-company group is better dealt with by a non-professional. The 'social group' should draw up a number of aims before it sets out and some such aims can be considered under the following areas:

1. Social skills training

What, if any, deficits are the group showing in the way of social skills? Events which can cater for the recognition of social etiquette and the 'normalised' patterns of behaviour which some activities require.

2. Assertion training

Assertion training can be used where group members feel that they are reticent or avoid situations which require some degree of positiveness.

The same is true of situations which require some form of modification of an over-enthusiastic participation in events which causes an 'arm's length' response from other participants.

3. Confrontation techniques

The problems and sensitivities of confrontation situations can be sorted out in a role-play format and may provide a certain amount of armour to those who are vulnerable in such settings.

4. Personal interaction

For those who are incapable of intimate interaction with other people the root cause can often be lack of practice or an unsureness of what is expected in such situations. Insights given into these areas can be helpful in socialising techniques.

The 'social group' can consider one or all of these areas. There are possibly other items which have not been mentioned here, all of which should have a positive contribution to make towards the 'social person' and how he can best be helped towards leading a fuller life.

The membership of the group requires some flexibility as the exclusion of members' friends and family may detract from its usefulness. The starting line for the group can be unambitious and cater for people whom the community psychiatric nurse may come across while working in the community. People often express an inability to go out or mix with people, or a fragmentation of some area of their social selves. The mere bringing together of individuals is, in itself, a therapeutic move. From such humble beginnings it is possible to move into more constructed areas of care. The role of the community psychiatric nurse in such a setting will require modification as time goes on. Such groups as this require a tremendous amount of effort to get them off the ground. The very fact of members attending such a group will produce problems of motivation and commitment among members initially and the community psychiatric nurse may well have to carry the group in the early stages.

The use of such a group will provide a medium through which it is possible to cater for several individuals at once. This will mean more time available to the community psychiatric nurse in the long run which can be used for more individual activities with other people.

Case study of sociotherapy

Mr C was a young man of 23 living at home with his mother. He had been diagnosed as schizophrenic at the age of 19 and had been in hospital on three occasions for two months at each admission. He was living the life of a hermit within the house and his mother had asked the consultant to 'try and gee him up a bit' and the consultant had duly passed on this task to the community psychiatric nurse. The community psychiatric nurse had visited on a number of occasions, and after lengthy discussions with Mr C and his mother, she decided that his reclusive habits were due to his complete inability to mix with other people and indulge in conversation naturally. Mr C expressed a wish to lead a fuller life. A role play situation was adopted by the community psychiatric nurse on future visits and Mr C was asked to perform social functions such as making tea and initiating conversation. This was fairly easily accomplished within the home setting and it was decided to take this into a more natural setting. The community psychiatric nurse was already running a small social-skills-training-group at a local church hall and the community psychiatric nurse took Mr C along to meet the other members. The group was given the power of its own decision making and programmes and Mr C was taken care of by one of the other members. After a number of sessions with the group, Mr C was able to attend on a number of social occasions and made some rather tentative relationships within the group. He never showed any inclination towards self-motivation other than on this one night per week.

Comments. This very familiar case of social disability because of lack of opportunities or inability to function is all too common. While this man could have been said to have achieved very little it could also be argued that his quality of life had been improved by a small percentage, not at the request of the consultant or by his mother, but because he himself had expressed a wish to do it. One can also add that his, admittedly tentative, contact with the group may have helped others within that group—and that is the essence of sociotherapy: using the group for the group!

SECTION B

In this section we must turn our attention to those behavioural sciences which seek to give explanations and provide insights into the context in which community psychiatric nursing is practised, viz. the community/society.

Sociology

Community psychiatric nurses are in varying degrees away from what is at one and the same time their protection and also their mentor i.e. the parent institution—the hospital. The fact that they are freed in this way naturally means that they are brought into contact in their daily work with society at large. So, whereas social psychology and often social psychiatry tend to concentrate on the person as an individual human being, sociology and medical sociology look at the person as one who has sets of rights, obligations and needs because of the particular position occupied within society. In order to understand the behaviour of any particular individual, therefore, one must have some knowledge of how society is structured and also how certain social institutions operate within the framework of society. Sociology is at one and the same time very abstract in the nature of its theorising, and very concrete in its applications to social situations. In order not to be left in any doubt as to the importance of sociology on our everyday lives one need only heed the writings of Emile Durkheim(56) one of the founding fathers of sociology. In two of his great works *Suicide* (1897) and *The Rules of Sociological Method* (1901) he showed the importance of the social context in determining how an individual thinks, feels and acts, and concluded that we do what we do because of the society in which we live and not because of the sort of people we are.

So sociology operates at a 'macro' level of analysis and being a very theoretical discipline it deals in variables: age, sex, class, race, religion, status, culture and so on. If a sociologist wants to examine some phenomenon, e.g. health/illness, he will tend to look at it in terms of the above and/or other variables—will collect and analyse data on the relationships between the phenomenon (independent variable) and each of its dependent variables (age, sex, etc.)—will present findings often statistical in nature—and will make recommendations which he hopes will be implemented. New phenomena may emerge giving rise to a need for more theorising and investigation and thus the cycle from theory to practice is completed and abstract thought takes on concrete form.

It is clearly right outside the scope of a text like this to look in any detail at the substantive areas of sociology. The sole concern of this section is to show the importance of sociology in the scheme of things in which we, as community psychiatric nurses operate—the less the social framework is recognised and understood, the more intangible becomes the social behaviour taking place within it.

In order to appreciate the place of sociology in the scheme of things one need only glance at journal articles bearing on community psychiatry in general, particularly during the last ten years. There one may see repeated discussion of topics which are in essence germane to sociology. The following examples—just a tiny sample from both sides of the Atlantic—serve to illustrate the point.

1. In 1967, Baggott(57), in discussing the role of the hospital nurse in the wider psychiatric service, focuses attention on the importance of re-socialisation and the need for nurses to learn a new therapeutic role

(Smith(58) has an interesting section on the former in his recent book).

2. In 1968, Green(59), in describing the community psychiatric nursing service at Moorhaven Hospital in Devon, spells out various aspects of the nurse's role complement, viz.:

the clinical role;
the team-member role;
the supportive role;
the preventive role;
the consultative role.

3. In 1969, Mechanic(60) talks about sociological issues in mental health and in discussing the question of using an educational model rather than a medical model in mental health raises many topics fundamental to sociology:

deviance;
labelling;
stigma;
social contexts;
social adaptation;
social change.

4. In 1970, Christman(61) noted the part which politics plays in the provision of mental health services.

5. In 1971, Wagenfeld(62) (see the reference list for Chapter 2 concerning this article) discusses the primary prevention of mental illness from a sociological perspective which includes an examination of community mental health *vis-à-vis* poverty and racism, and ideological considerations.

6. In 1972, Stobie and Hopkins(63), in describing the Dingleton community nurse, dwell on the question of the team approach with all that that entails for the status of the respective team members and also on their role in crisis intervention situations.

7. In 1973, Maxwell(64), in looking at the health visitor's role in community psychiatry, analyses it in terms of her traditional functions.

8. In 1974, Williams(65), writing about community psychiatric nursing in Canada, draws attention to the importance of cultural differences between communities. (This of course is quite apparent in the north of Canada to which he was referring. What may not be so apparent in a high-density population area like the U.K. is the fact that cultural differences—quite apart from those presented by immigrant families—do exist and need to be borne in mind; this brings the concept of 'class' into the discussion.)

9. In 1975, Pilisuk(66) discusses the very interesting question of social control through the agency of technical jargon in the field of

mental health. The article is full of sociological jibes directed at 'mystifying semantics', 'elite educated mandarins' and 'therapists masquerading behind intellectual stereotypes'—a quite splendid essay!

10. In 1976, Pinkerton(67), in looking at paediatric psychiatry, examines the importance of the family in preserving a stable, balanced way of life which is conducive to mental health. Parental attitudes are a crucial factor in the prevention of mental illness. (Interestingly enough in the same month of the same year—January 1976—but this time on the other side of the Atlantic, Cohler et al.(68) compare child care attitudes and adaptation to the maternal role among mentally ill and mentally well mothers and note that 'Mentally ill mothers were found to believe less in the importance of developing a reciprocal mother-child relationship or in differentiating between own needs and those of the child and were more likely to deny ambivalent feelings towards child care'!)

11. In 1977, Opit(69) looks at the economic factors involved in the provision of domiciliary care.

The reader will thus realise from this very small selection of journal articles the importance of a knowledge of sociology for the community psychiatric nurse today. Such knowledge enables the practitioner to view the structure of society through a knowledge of its institutions and artefacts and consequently to understand the constraints it imposes in ordinary, everyday life.

Medical sociology

David Robinson(70) indicates quite nicely the scope of medical sociology:

> That man is a social animal means quite simply that his actions cannot be adequately described, much less explained, without understanding and making reference to the social and cultural situation within which he operates. The sociological enterprise is geared to explaining actions in particular social situations through gaining an understanding of how the persons involved in that situation see and interpret the world around them. The 'medical' sociologist is merely a sociologist whose particular concern is medical and related situations.

The sociological perspective in what we may call the 'medical world' for the sake of simplicity, shows itself in a number of areas of interest:

the sick role;

relationships — doctor-patient ⎫
            nurse-patient ⎬ the concept of status
            nurse-doctor ⎭

professions: the study of medicine, nursing;

the concept of professionalisation;

the professions and bureaucracy;
the hospital as a complex organisation;
social class and health;
social causes of disease;
culture and health;
the organisation and delivery of health care;
iatrogenesis.

This is by no means an inclusive list, but does indicate perhaps the main areas of interest in this field.

There is, of course, almost always a fundamental problem to be overcome when introducing doctors/nurses/paramedics to sociology: medicine/nursing and sociology are quite different areas of knowledge —the one being mainly factual and practice-based disciplines, the other being a theoretical orientation which may be brought to bear on society as represented in any of its institutions. Socialised as they are—as men/women of action—nurses/doctors all too often tend to think of sociology as rather vague and ineffectual. Were the reader to think thus, he would be doing himself as a practitioner and all potential patients/clients a grave disservice. As Tuckett(71) notes:

> Through greater sociological understanding many clinical judgements may be made more rationally, much of the frustration in present-day practice may be overcome; the behaviour of patients, of colleagues and of large organisations may be better appreciated, and the doctor may be able to exercise the therapeutic skills he has learnt in other parts of his training more effectively for the benefit of his patients.

These words might well have been directed at nurses as well; and if they hold good for nurses/doctors in general medicine then they hold doubly good for those engaged in looking after the mentally ill—especially those working in the community where a deeper knowledge and understanding of society's institutions is required for effective practice.

As has been stressed above, it is no part of this book to delve into the substantive parts of particular behavioural sciences in any depth: they are mentioned to illustrate their relevance to the community psychiatric nurse of today and it is hoped that areas of particular interest to the reader will be followed up via the bibliography at the end of the chapter.

In order to underpin the significance of medical sociology for the community psychiatric nurse there follows, as previously from both sides of the Atlantic, a short selection of journal articles illustrating the impact of medical sociological ideas on the practice of community psychiatry/psychiatric nursing:

1. In 1967, Herman and Swank(72) discuss the unifying of hospital

and community efforts in the delivery of a comprehensive mental health care programme.

2. In 1968, Arafeh *et al.*(73) look at the same kind of problem—linking the hospital and community efforts in the delivery of care for psychiatric patients. A more comprehensive article which gives some useful insights into the planning of such programmes and into hospitals as institutions.

3. In 1969, Crossley and Denmark(74) provide an interesting account of some social causes of disease in their study of the psychiatric morbidity of a Salvation Army hostel.

4. In 1970, Mesnikoff(75) in evaluating some dilemmas in community psychiatry casts some interesting sidelights on:

the professions and bureaucracy;
the patient and bureaucracy;
social class and health;
the organisation of health care.

5. In 1971, Gottesfeld(76) describes an information system for assessing community mental health projects which illustrates both the importance of research in the monitoring of the delivery and extension of health care, and the importance of having a system for evaluating the particular research projects.

6. In 1972, Arnhoff(77) gives a very comprehensive account of the relationships between manpower issues and the theory and practice of mental health. He points out the need for sub-goal specification in the organisation and delivery of health care and sounds a warning against the blanket use of statistics as a planning tool.

7. In 1973, Haldane and Lindsey(78) focus attention on child and family psychiatry and stress the need for the relevant professions to work together to achieve an integrated service. This in turn means looking at the various professions invlolved, identifying the nature of each and indicating ways of operating on an interdisciplinary basis.

8. In 1974, Leopoldt, Hopkins and Overall(79) describe an on-going experimental attachment scheme in Oxford, and compare the results of a number of surveys done on different phases of the attachment. It throws light on the problems of liaising between hospital and the primary health care team and makes recommendations about integration and the team work approach.

9. In 1975, Christie(80) discusses community mental health from the standpoint of approaches to it—in this case the 'service' and 'organisational' approaches. This is a nice philosophical discussion which perhaps best illustrates the nature of the sociological approach—that it is a science of ideas which, brought to bear on particular aspects of practice, can be very fruitful.

10. In 1976, White and Hunter(81) examine critically the use of non-medical manpower in community psychiatry—the use of the non-medical therapist. Their cost-effectiveness is looked at as also are the positive and negative aspects of the available alternatives.

11. In 1977, Donnelly(82) looks at the area of professional relationships in community psychiatric nursing: in this particular article the roles of the social worker and the community psychiatric nurse are examined.

It will readily be appreciated that medical sociology has much to offer to the developing field of community psychiatric nursing. Workers in this field are brought into daily contact with man as a social animal—less medicalised, less labelled, less stigmatised than the patient in the hospital. They encounter illness less as a bureaucratised figment of medical imagination, more on its own terms as a bio-social phenomenon. To meet it on its own terms and thus be of help in alleviating it, they must add the 'social' component to their existing medical/nursing stock-in-trade. The one sure way of achieving this is by drawing on the general concepts that go to make up the field of sociology and the particular themes which are dealt with in the specialised field of medical sociology.

SECTION C

In sections A and B of this chapter we have looked respectively at the behavioural sciences which impinge on the practice and context of community psychiatric nursing. Community psychiatric nursing may only be so arbitrarily divided for the purposes of exposition and discussion—in real life the fabric of the field is woven with the behavioural strands already mentioned, plus others like psychology, social administration, education, in such a way as to come to terms with the real needs and problems of a community. In order to illustrate how an area of community psychiatric nursing is shot through with allusions and references to the behavioural sciences, there follows a discussion of the relationship between community psychiatric nursing, mental handicap and the behavioural sciences.

Discussion

The nurse will require a knowledge of the effects of definition on the service provided and on the incidence and prevalence rates of mental handicap in different social situations. The number of mentally handicapped people in the community is not known with any degree of certainty. Various surveys from that of the Wood Committee 1929(83) to the Tizard London survey(84) and the Birch survey of 1962(85) arrive at figures around 3.7 per 1000 severely subnormal, as Tizard(84) was so careful to state—'of severely subnormal children of school age'. From the normal curve of distribution there would be 100 000 mentally retarded people in this country. Services are planned on the basis of 5/1000. The differences between true-ascertained and administrative figures are an indication of the number of families within the community who are left unsupported. When the prevalence rates for the subnormal or moderately handicapped are considered even less is known as so much depends on community tolerance. The number of people who may be considered mentally handicapped varies under different social situations. In times of high unemployment or high levels of inflation the mentally handicapped are more likely to surface as a result of redundancy or budgetry problems. As Lorna Wing(86) has shown the additional problems of identification arise as people who might be regarded as of sufficiently low intelligence to be called mentally handicapped are unknown to the authorities, yet people who have intelligence levels within the normal range come into contact with the mental handicap agencies.

Here the social definition of Dexter(87) has its attractions—the notion that the problems of the mentally handicapped stem from the attitudes of people to mental handicap rather than from the handicap itself. Coupled to this one might consider—if the criterion for mental handicap is social incompetence—is whether the person be so labelled when he becomes socially competent.

Whilst considering the prevalence rates of mental handicap and the interesting revelations of Birch(85) of the differences in prevalence rates of the mildly subnormal in the various social classes—predominating in social class 5, absent in social class 1—there are a number of explanations, the truth being that it is multifactorial. The so-called subcultural group results from assortive mating where people of low intelligence marry and beget children who themselves are 'not very bright'. Yet by the phenomenon of regression to the mean these children tend to be more intelligent than their parents, and likely, because of this differential, to be under-estimated. Some of the cause of underfunctioning must thereby be cultural and hence amenable to education if the family is supported early. We may not be able to do any better than our genes allow but we can, and frequently do, worse. This area of positive help does not appear to be currently part of any family support system with the emphasis at present being on the severely handicapped and their families. In this case the need for help is more obvious and for the family more pressing, yet the less intelligent families who require services are unlikely to be aware of the availability buy appropriate clothing or food, and fail to stimulate at the appropriate level. It is the families who most require the services who are the least likely to be aware of their existence!

Besides the differing prevalence rates in social groups the nurse needs to be aware of the differing effects of mental handicap on the family. Children with Downs syndrome in institutional care are over-represented from social groups 1 and 5, but for different reasons. In social group 1 placement results from dashed hopes and failed expectations. From birth, often before, the life and career of the child is foreseen—following the family business or profession—marriage, yet these hopes fade when the handicap is diagnosed. Therein lies a crisis. From social class 5 the problem is not so much with personal expectations projected through the child, (the child as extension of the parent), but the reasons are more likely to be economic. The difficulty of managing on low wages and poor budgeting is highlighted by a child who wears out clothes, shoes, and furniture at an accelerated rate.

Nurse must be aware of the effects on the family from initial suspicion through diagnosis and the various family crises—moving house, illness, school, adolescence, occupation, marriage, and place-ment that will affect the family with a handicapped member differently as a result of the handicap. In this context the nurse must be aware of the observed effects on families, not those effects one would expect to meet. Being told that your child is handicapped is the greatest cause of distress in a life full of stress. The most commonly reported reaction is that of grief or chronic sorrow. So often one hears the term 'guilt' in relation to having a handicapped child. Lay persons and professionals alike attempt to influence the parent into a position of guilt: 'Did you feel guilty?' to which the answer is often affirmative; but is that politeness or the difficulty of labelling an abstract feeling? The tendency to label parents as anxiety-laden and guilt-ridden is indeed unfortunate, for in truth there is no adequate way that the family can show that they are not guilty, any actions being taken as evidence of guilt rather than its absence. Although a handicapped child will have effects on the family of an emotional, social, and economic nature, one should ascertain to what extent emotional disturbances, or behavioural observations, are common in the normal population. (Note the findings of Holt in the Sheffield survey 1957(88) who found quarrelling in 6 per cent of families with a handicapped member.)

The nurse will require a knowledge of crisis intervention theory, not just intervening to give help in whatever form, but to be aware of the need to consider not only the appropriateness and effectiveness of the family's coping skills, but how much help of what kind, when, in order, that the episode becomes a learning experience helping the family to develop their coping techniques rather than a dependency on any helping agency. The family should be more able to deal with a subsequent crisis of a similar nature.

The nurse/client relationship in the community is of a different order than in the traditional hospital situation and more akin to the more liberal progressive ethos. The concepts of personal boundaries and professional distancing is here relevant. A feature of institutions of all types is the distance the caring keep themselves from the cared-for, especially in the social emotional spheres and often physically also. The distance is controlled by the staff who project their personal professional boundaries by a number of techniques involving both verbal and non-verbal communication. The client is not, however, in a position to establish an invisible personal boundary. The nurse has the privilege of invading the privacy of the patient, controlling his environment and his behaviour, even though it is to all intents and purposes the patients' home and not that of the nurse: the role-relationship determines the behaviour of the incumbents. Where the commune ethos is in evidence with all-helping-all this is less in evidence and may in fact be absent. The personal boundaries in this situation arise by mutual understanding between the parties. Professional distancing is as unwelcome as it is unnecessary.

Within the home a professional relationship is appropriate yet it is the nurse who is on unfamiliar ground. Here the family is in greater control of boundaries and their privacy, no more important than that of the hospitalised patient (by that one means that the privacy of the hospitalised patient is important though largely neglected) is much more sacrosanct. The nurse must be prepared to roll up sleeves and not only offer advice but give practical expert help within the home—not only telling, but showing parents how they can help in the care, assessment, treatment and education of their child.

The nurse will need to be aware of the professional current and past relationships and the advice given. Much of the parents coping strategies may be based on, or arise as a result of information given by other people both professional and non-professional. Under-achieving, a common enough phenomenon, arises because people are not appropriately stimulated as a result of our expectations of them being set at too low a level. Such advice as parents are given is largely discouraging rather than encouraging. Some groups of enthusiastic parents encourage one another to develop their children, some seek progress through the patterning procedures of the Doman Delacato(89) system of stimulation. Mentally handicapped people require appropriate stimulation, and within the family is the best place and the best people to undertake the stimulation, but they must not be ill advised, given false hopes and misleading reassurances, but be given encouraging realistic information and guidance from experienced people with true empathy.

Professionals have for too long and for too often encouraged families to treat their members with mental retardation (families do not use the term 'mental subnormality') as children. Some of the publicity material from the National Society for Mentally Handicapped Children follows a similar vein—'children who never grow'. An awareness of normal human development is not only useful as an assessment and treatment tool in terms of sensory motor conceptual development, but also in terms of the socialisation process through which children go, involving learning society's rules and behaving in a socially acceptable way appropriate to one's age and development. The mentally retarded should not be allowed to circumvent or ignore social conventions on account of their handicap. Sitting on laps at 18 years of age is not abnormal, yet one does not do it indiscriminately, and to complete strangers. Mentally handicapped people may fail to learn the right meaning of events, symbols, or things of social significance but could this be on account of inappropriate teaching rather than defective learning. The handicapped person should be allowed, nay encouraged, to develop socially in accordance with their age and maturation. It is common to transfer the dependent child to the dependent adult without allowing them to go through the intermediate stage of transition we call adolescence.

This is the time when people not designated as handicapped go through problems of identity of developing their individualism rather than the carbon copy of parental dress and attitudes. It is a time when interest in the opposite sex goes through a more intimate finding out and knowing stage, and may end in the 'child' leaving the parental home. Leaving a home amicably is not uncommon during the later stages of adolescence.

Development of the personhood of the person is just as important for the handicapped. They too need to go through the adolescent phase of transition away from home: they too must be given the opportunity to become aware of the fulfilment that love can bring, and also the heartaches and distress that relationships can engender when they break up. The handicapped too must be given the opportunity for marriage, and be adequately prepared for the event.

Moving away from home to alternative care may also be appropriate in late adolescence. Here the community nurse must be aware of the alternative patterns of residential care, and the quality of care that is given. Where the nurse has responsibility for homes within the community this is the more important. The nurse must be aware of the work of Miller and Gwynne(90), Tizard and Grad(91), King and Rayne(92) and Maureen Oswin(93) and develop a liberal and humane approach to care. Recently a woman of 40 was admitted to a hostel in order to acclimatise her to residential care in preparation for the day when such care would be necessary. The insistence of the hostel warden that somebody should sit in the bathroom when she had a bath (she had been bathing herself for 30 years by her own testimony), and his lack of regard for her privacy—going into her bedroom whilst she was in her underclothes—has made her resolve not to go into a hostel. The nurses must come down from their professional plinth and stand or fall on their expertise of helping the handicapped rather than on their hierarchical pose which is beginning to fool no-one.

'Normalisation', which is a word which competes with 'community care' for the cliche of the decade award, is nevertheless an important concept in the care of the handicapped: with the implications of the normal rights of citizenship, the pattern of life of the mainstream of society whilst acknowledging the appropriateness or otherwise of the concept for the handicapped in terms of their tendency to anticipate failure rather than success, their emotional instability and the tendency to collapse under pressure. Whilst not dogmatically following the advocates of normalisation the nurse needs to be aware of its implications for the handicapped, always remembering that normalisation applies to the family as well.

Perception is a concept with which the nurse must have more than a passing knowledge. It occurs in different areas with different perspectives, yet pervades the whole scene. It is an important conceptual development in the learning of the handicapped, developing the ability to perceive shapes, moving from simple to more complex shapes, leading indirectly to the 'social-sight vocabulary'. It is a phenomenon of which the nurse must be aware in the advising of parents such that if the information is incomplete the learner will fill the gap, probably inappropriately, or if the advice is confused or lacking in meaning for the listener, they will either forget or make the information make sense to themselves, which may be different from the way it was intended. Perception from a sociological viewpoint can be seen as giving meaning to our lives, and therefore happiness, the quality of which depends to a large extent on the meaning we project into our existence and our environment and the interpretation we place upon our lives.

The attitudes we adopt to life depend on this interpretation. The nurse must be aware that the quality of life is so dependent on interpretation and that the interpretation of the nurse may be different from the interpretation of the family, and that each may affect the meaning the other extracts from the situation. One here hesitates to use the word 'problem', as this tends to anticipate the situation and therein lies the problem. Self-fulfilling prophesies fit neatly into this category. One must be wary of the effect of labelling or perception and hence the meaning attached to incidents or people. Expectations influence events such that the events match expectations more closely. We anticipate the actions and behaviour of people according to labels attached to them. Downs syndrome sufferers are happy, musical, friendly and severely subnormal—but do we adversely influence their behaviour by our expectations and our limited perception? Epileptics are seen as fickle, bad tempered, strangers to the truth. The stereotype becomes a consistently applied label, influences our expectation and their perceived performance. Observers note phenomena that reinforce their preconceived notion, ignoring information that does not fit. People are people, and although it is necessary for orderly existence that we adopt strategies based on familiarity and expectations, the nurse needs to be aware of the inherent dangers attached to these processes.

Information not received as intended, illustrates a failure of communication—another field of which nurses must be aware.

Communication is a two-way process involving a sender who encodes a message to be transmitted to a receiver who in turn decodes the message. Communication is effective if the message is received as the sender had intended. The sender requires to interpret the effect of his message on the receiver. The community nurse needs to be particularly aware of the need for effective communication with the client. He must be sure that the language both in style and content is capable of being understood by the family. The nurse must have an awareness of non-verbal and verbal communication, to develop a sensitivity to cues indicating the relationships within the family. Communication operates at a number of different levels. It may be a superficial open level with feelings hidden. Within the relationships that constitute communication each attempts to get the other to reveal what they would prefer to conceal. Each is also attempting to get the other to become aware of attributes obvious to the observer but of which the person is himself unaware. Other factors affecting behaviour, and hence communication, will have unconscious motivation of which both participants are unaware. The community nurse must be aware of these various elements of communication in order to be an effective practititioner in the community.

REFERENCES

1. Berelson, B. and Steiner, G. A. (1964) *Human Behaviour: An Inventory of Scientific Findings*. New York: Harcourt.
2. Bowart, W. (1978) *Operation Mind Control*. Glasgow: Fontana.
3. Barton, R. (1976) *Institutional Neurosis*. 3rd edn. Bristol: Wright.
4. Goffman, E. (1961) *Asylums*. Harmondsworth: Penguin Books Limited.
5. Frost, M. (1972) Institutionalisation of mental nurses. *British Hospital Journal and Social Service Review*. February 5th.
6. Mead, G. H. (1934) *Mind, Self and Society from the Standpoint of a Social Behaviourist*. Chicago: University of Chicago Press.
7. Moreno, J. L. (1934) *Who Shall Survive?* Washington: Nervous and Mental Disease Publishing Company.
8. Linton, R. (1945) *The Cultural Background of Personality*. New York: Appleton-Century-Crofts.
9. Biddle, B. J. and Thomas, E. J. (Eds) (1966) *Role Theory – Concepts and Research*. New York: Wiley.
10. Secord, P. F. and Backman, C. W. (1964) *Social Psychology*. New York: McGraw-Hill.
11. Goffman, E. (1959) *The Presentation of Self in Everyday Life*. New York: Doubleday Anchor.
12. Briggs Report (1972) *Report of the Committee on Nursing*. H.M.S.O. Cmnd 5115.
13. Argyle, M. (1967) *The Psychology of Interpersonal Behaviour*. Harmondsworth: Penguin Books Limited.
14. Peplau, H. E. (1952) *Interpersonal relations in nursing*. New York: Putnam's Sons.
    Peplau, H. E. (1966) Talking with patients and Interpersonal techniques: the crux of psychiatric nursing. In *Psychiatric Nursing*, **1**. Mereness, D. Dubuque, Iowa: Brown.
15. Actschul, A. (1972) *Patient/Nurse Interaction*. Edinburgh: Churchill Livingstone.
16. Trower, P., Bryant, B. and Argyle, M. (1978) *Social Skills and Mental Health*. London: Methuen.
17. Argyle, M. (1973) *Social Interaction*. London: Tavistock.
18. Skinner, B. F. (1957) *Verbal Behaviour*. New York: Appleton-Century-Crofts.
19. Bell, R. T. (1976) *Sociolinguistics*. London: Batsford.
20. Davis, A. J. (1966) The skills of communication. In *Psychiatric Nursing*. Vol. One. Mereness, D. (Ed) Dubuque, Iowa: Brown.
21. Ruesch, J. (1967) The role of communication in therapeutic transactions. In *The Human Dialogue*. Matson, F. W. and Montagu, A. (eds) New York: The Free Press.
22. Eldred, S. H. (1966) Improving nurse/patient communications. In *Psychiatric Nursing*. Vol. One. Mereness, D. (ed) Dubuque, Iowa: Brown.
23. Greenhill, M. H. (1966) Interviewing with a purpose. In *Psychiatric Nursing*. Vol. One. Mereness, D. (ed) Dubuque, Iowa: Brown.
24. Carr, P. J. (1979) 'To describe the role of the nurse working in a psychiatric unit which is situated in a district general hospital complex.' Unpublished Ph.D. Thesis, University of Manchester.
25. Laing, R. D. (1977) *Do You Love Me?* Harmondsworth: Penguin Books Limited.
26. Orford, J. (1976) *The Social Psychology of Mental Disorder*. Harmondsworth: Penguin Books Limited.
27. Rogers, C. R. (1969) *Encounter Groups*. Harmondsworth: Penguin Books Limited.
28. Hollander, E. P. (1967) *Principles and Methods of Social Psychology*. New York: Oxford University Press.

29. Taylor, D. A. and Kleinhans, B. (1976), Group development and structure. In *Social psychology*. Seidenberg and Snadowsky, A. New York: The Free Press.
30. Bales, R. F. (1970) *Personality and Interpersonal Behaviour*. New York: Holt, Rinehart & Winston.
31. Steiner, I. D. (1972) *Group Process and Productivity*. New York: Academic Press.
32. Kleinhans, B. and Taylor, D. A. (1976) Group processes, productivity, and leadership. In *Social Psychology*. Seidenberg, B. and Snadowsky, A. New York: The Free Press.
33. Slater, P. E. (0000) *The Pursuit of Loneliness: American Culture at the Breaking Point*. Boston: Beacon Press.
34. Gahagan, J. (1975) *Interpersonal and Group Behaviour*. London: Methuen.
35. Klein, J. (1961) *Working with Groups*. London: Hutchinson University Library.
36. Siegler, M. and Osmond, H. (1974) *Models of Madness, Models of Medicine*. New York: Macmillan Publishing Co. Ltd.
37. Cooper, D. (1970) *Psychiatry and Anti-Psychiatry*. St. Albans: Paladin.
38. Toffler, A. (1971) *Future Shock*. London: Pan Books Limited.
39. Szasz, T. S. (1972) *The Myth of Mental Illness*. St. Albans: Paladin.
    Szasz, T. S. (1974) *Ideology and Insanity*. Harmondsworth: Penguin Books Limited.
    Szasz, T. S. (1971) *The Manufacture of Madness*. London: Routledge and Kegan Paul.
40. Watson, J. B. (1966) Behaviourism and the concept of mental disease, *J. Philos. Psychol. Scient. Meth.*, **13**, 587–97.
41. Pavlov, I, P. (1932) Neuroses in men and animals. *Journal of the American Medical Association*, **99**, 1012–13.
    Pavlov, I. P. *Conditioned Reflexes and Psychiatry*. New York: International University Press.
42. Lindsley, O. R. and Skinner, B. F. (1954) A method for the experimental analysis of the behaviour of psychiatric patients, *American Psychology*, **9**, 419–20.
43. Eysenck, H. J. (1960) *Behaviour Therapy and the Neuroses*. London: Pergamon.
    Eysenck, H. J. and Rachman, S. (1965) *The Causes and Cures of Neuroses*. London: Routledge and Kegan Paul.
44. Yates, A. J. (1970) *Behaviour Therapy*. New York: Wiley.
45. Wolpe, J. (1973) *The Practice of Behaviour Therapy*. New York: Pergamon.
46. Orwell, G. (1954) *Nineteen Eighty-Four*. Harmondsworth: Penguin Books Limited (Modern Classics).
47. Kreeger, L. (1974) Psychotherapy in the past, present and future. In *Psychotherapy Today*. Varma, V. (ed) London: Constable.
48. Freud, S. (1954) *The Interpretation of Dreams*. New York: Basic Books Limited.
49. Walrond-Skinner, S. (1976) *Family Therapy*. London: Routledge and Kegan Paul.
50. Freedman, A. M., Kaplan, H. I. and Sadock, B. J. (1976) *Modern Synopsis of Comprehensive Textbook of Psychiatry/11*. Baltimore: The Williams & Wilkins Co.
51. Jones, M. (1952) *Social Psychiatry*. London: Tavistock.
52. Jahoda, M. (1958) *Current Concepts of Positive Mental Health*. New York: Basic Books.
53. Scheff, T. J. (1966) *Being Mentally Ill: A Sociological Theory*. Chicago: Aldine.
54. Becker, H. S. (1963) *Outsiders: Studies in the Sociology of Behaviour*. New York: The Free Press.
55. Clare, A. (1976) *Psychiatry in Dissent*. London: Tavistock.
56. Durkheim, E. (1947) *The Division of Labour in Society*. New York: Macmillan.
    Durkheim, E. (1950) *The Rules of Sociological Method*. Chicago: Chicago University Press.
    Durkheim, E. (1951) *Suicide: A Study in Sociology*. Free Press of Glencoe.

57. Baggott, E. (1967) Role of the hospital nurse in the wider psychiatric service, *Nursing Times*, **63**, No. 30, 993–94.
58. Smith, J. P. (1976) *Sociology and Nursing*. Edinburgh: Churchill Livingstone.
59. Greene, J. (1968) The psychiatric nurse in the community nursing service, *Int. Journal of Nursing Studies*, **5**, 175–84.
60. Mechanic, D. (1969) Sociological issues in mental health, *Progress in Community Health*, **1**.
61. Christman, L. (1970) Continuity of psychiatric care: the present model, *Perspectives in Psychiatric Care*, **VIII**, No. 2.
62. Wagenfield, M. O. (1972) The primary prevention of mental illness: a sociological perspective, *Journal of Health and Social Behaviour*.
63. Stobie, E. G. and Hopkins, D. H. G. (1972) Crisis intervention (1 and 2), *Nursing Times Occasional Papers*, October 26th and November 2nd.
64. Maxwell, A. (1973) The health visitor's role in community psychiatry, *Nursing Mirror*, **139**, 74–6.
65. Williams, R. (1974) Teamwork, the key to community psychiatric nursing, *Canadian Journal of Psychiatric Nursing*, **15**, 15–17.
66. Pilisuk, M. (1975) Mental health mystification and social control, *American Journal of Orthopsychiatry*, **45**, No. 3, 14–19.
67. Pinkerton, P. (1976) Paediatric psychiatry, *Nursing Mirror*, January 15th.
68. Cohler, B. J., Grunebaum, H. U., Weiss, J. L., Hartman, C. R. and Gallant, D. H. (1976) Child care attitudes and adaptations to the maternal role among mentally ill and well mothers, *American Journal of Orthopsychiatry*, **46**, No. 1, 123–34.
69. Opit, L. J. (1977) Domiciliary care for the elderly sick—economy or neglect? *British Medical Journal*, **1**, 30–33.
70. Robinson, D. (1973) *Patients, Practitioners and Medical Care*. London: Heinemann.
71. Tuckett, D. (Ed). (1976) *An Introduction to Medical Sociology*. London: Tavistock.
72. Herman, A. and Swank, L. (1967) Unifying hospital and community efforts, *Hospital and Commun. Psych.*, **18**, No. 3, 83–4.
73. Arafeh, M. K., Fumiatti, E. K., Gregory, M. E., Reilly, M. and Wolfe, I. S. (1968) Linking hospital and community care for psychiatric patients, *American Journal of Nursing*, **68**, No. 5, 1050–56.
74. Crossley, B. and Denmark, J. C. (1969) Community care—a study of the morbidity of a salvation army hostel, *British Journal of Sociology*, **20**, 443–49.
75. Mesnikoff, A. M. (1970) Dilemmas in community psychiatry. *International Journal of Psychiatry*, **9**, 312–18.
76. Gottesfeld, H. (1971) An information system for assessing community mental health projects, *Hospital and Commun. Psych.*, **22**, 14–16.
77. Arnhoff, F. N. (1972) Manpower needs, resources and innovations, *Progress in Community Mental Health*, **2**, 35–61.
78. Haldane, J. D. and Lindsay, S. F. (1973) Child and family psychiatry in an integrated child health services, *Health Bulletin*, **31**, No. 2, 79–85.
79. Leopoldt, H., Hopkins, H. and Overall, R. (1974) A critical review of experimental psychiatric nurse attachment in Oxford, *Practice Team*, **39**, 2–6.
80. Christie, J. R. (1975) The community and mental health, *Canadian Welfare*, **511**, No. 6, 5–8.
81. White, N. F. and Hunter, D. G. (1976) Instead of psychiatrists: a critical look at non-medical manpower, *Canadian Journal of Public Health*, **67**, 15–20.
82. Donnelly, G. (1977) Relationships: the social worker and psychiatric community nurse, *Nursing Mirror*, September 22nd.
83. Lewis, E. O. (1929) *The Report of the Mental Deficiency Committee being a Joint Committee of the Board of Education and Board of Control: Part IV – Report of an investigation into the incidence of mental deficiency in six areas, 1925-1927*. London: H.M.S.O.

84. Tizard, J. (1964) *Community Services for the mentally handicapped*. London: Oxford University Press.
85. Birch, H. E., Richardson, S. A., Baird, D., Horobin, E. and Illsley, R. (1970) *Mental Subnormality in the Community: a Clinical and Epidemiologic study*. Baltimore: Williams and Wilkins.
86. Wing, L. (1971) Severely retarded children in a London area: prevalence and provision of services, *Psychol. Med.*, **1**, 405–415.
87. Dexter, L. A. (1958) *American Journal of Mental Deficiency*, **63**, 920–28.
88. Holt, K. S. (1958) The influence of a retarded child upon family limitations, *Paediatrics*, **22**, 744–55.
89. Doman, G. (1974) *What to do about your Brain Injured Child*. London: Jonathan Cape.
90. Miller, E. J. and Gwynne, G. V. (1972) *A Life Apart: A Report of a Pilot Study of Residential Institutions for the Physically Handicapped and Young Chronic Sick*. London: Tavistock.
91. Tizard, J. and Grad, J. C. (1961) *The Mentally Handicapped and their Families*. London: Oxford University Press.
92. King, R. D., Raynes, N. V. and Tizard, J. (1971) *Patterns of Residential Care*. London: Routledge and Kegan Paul.
93. Oswin, M. (1971) *The Empty Hours*. London: Allen Lane.

8

Community psychiatric nursing and the law: an outline

INTRODUCTION

The law has come to play an increasingly important part in the life of the health care practitioner and this is a trend which is likely to continue. It behoves all who work in the National Health Service to pay more attention to the legal aspects of their work—in this way will trouble be best avoided: 'forewarned is forearmed'!

The legal education of nurses is, generally speaking, woefully inadequate—it would be unfair, therefore, to single out psychiatric nurses in this respect. Having said that, however, let it also be noted that if any one group of nurses really needs to be aware of the legal implications of their work it is those who care for people who for one reason or another may act irrationally from time to time. Mental handicap nurses and psychiatric nurses deal with people who are often inherently unstable and the law quite rightly protects such unfortunate people. For practitioners working in such delicate areas not to know the main provisions of the law relating to their job is most unfortunate to say the least!

Community psychiatric nurses have the worst of all possible deals when it comes to the law. If ever one group of nurses could be said to be vulnerable in this area, then that group would, without any doubt, be community psychiatric nurses. This is so for the two following reasons:

1. they are dealing with disturbed people;
2. they are working in the community, away from the guardianship of that vast and watchful bureaucracy, the National Health Service, and thus likely to be 'on their own' in the event of anything untoward occurring: witnesses to events are likely to be on the patient's rather than the nurse's side.

Szasz(1) and Gostin(2) have written revealingly about the inadequacies of the law relating to the mentally ill—curtailment of rights, loss of freedoms, etc., and their words ring true. Little, however, has been said of the inadequacies of the law as it relates to mental handicap and psychiatric nurses—and for the reasons given above, those who work away from the institution are most at risk—but there can be no doubt whatever that in the face of allegations (of whatever sort, e.g. violence, sexual misconduct, theft) the nurse is *ipso facto* in an extremely vulnerable position.

The sources of English law
(N.B. the law referred to in this chapter is specifically English law. English law is the basis of the Anglo-American or 'common law' group of legal systems and applies in England and Wales and, for the most part, in Northern Ireland. Scots law belongs to a small group of 'mixed' legal systems which have their roots in both English and Roman law.)

The main sources of English law are the following:

1. legislation:
   statutes (Acts of Parliament);
   delegated legislation (statutory instruments, by-laws);
2. the common law:
   judge-made law based on the doctrine of judicial precedent;
3. equity:
   deriving from the Court of Chancery, but now just another branch of law dealing with trusts in the main;
4. European community law:
   The European Communities Act, 1972, became part of our legal framework when we became a member of the European Community on January 1st, 1973. It relates mainly, at the moment, to economic and social matters.

A glance at this list will be sufficient to show that we need only concern ourselves with (1) and (2): legislation and 'the common law'.

Branches of the English law
The two main branches are the following:

1. Criminal law:
   acts, attempts, incitements or conspiracies against the person, e.g. murder; against property, e.g. theft; or against the State, e.g. treason. Offences may be serious, that is 'indictable' (usually tried before judge and jury) or ordinary, that is 'summary' (usually tried before magistrates);
2. Civil law:
   the law of contract; the law of torts; the law of property; family law.

There are other less important branches of English law:

1. Administrative law;
2. Admiralty law;
3. Ecclesiastical law;
4. Industrial law;
5. Service law.

By much the greatest branch of English law is the civil law.

The layman may sometimes have difficulty in grasping the difference between the criminal and civil law because the distinction does not reside in the nature of the act or omission. Rather does it lie in what kind of proceedings may follow said act or omission: if criminal proceedings are instituted by the Crown then you stand accused of a criminal offence; if, however, an action is taken against you under private law, i.e. by some person or other (usually an injured party or his representative) then you are accused of some civil wrong-doing. So the same act can be both a crime and a civil wrong. Glanville Williams (3) gives a nice example to illustrate the point:

> Suppose that at the railway station I entrust my bag to someone who offers to carry it for rewards, and he runs off with it. He has committed the crime of theft and also two civil wrongs—the tort of conversion and breach of his contract with me to carry the bag safely. The result is that two sorts of legal proceedings can be taken against him: a prosecution for the crime, and a civil action for the tort and for the breach of contract.

Criminal and civil cases are tried in different courts. The courts with criminal jurisdiction are:

Magistrates' courts;
the Crown Court (for the more serious kind of offence);
the Court of Appeal (criminal division);
the House of Lords—a Law Lords Committee.

The courts with civil jurisdiction are:

magistrates courts (very limited jurisdiction);
county courts;
the High Court (for the more important kind of case);
the Court of Appeal (civil division);
the House of Lords—a Law Lords Committee.

The court system is more complicated than that, but these notes are a guide to the general layout of court business.

Activities in the criminal courts are referred to as prosecutions, and are of an 'accusatorial' nature. A prosecution is a contest between the Crown and the accused person (the defendant). Usually the police act as agents of the Crown in instituting proceedings, although some offences can only be prosecuted with the consent of the Attorney

General or the Director of Public Prosecutions. If the accused person is found guilty, the penalty is either of a custodial nature, i.e. imprisonment, or may be non-custodial e.g. fine, probation, 'binding over', conditional discharge. Additionally, for qualified nurses, i.e. registered or enrolled nurses, or for nurses in training, i.e. student/pupil nurses, there is the question of being reported to the statutory body—the General Nursing Council—if found guilty. The Home Secretary has a list of criteria which indicate which offences must be reported to statutory bodies—if a particular offence comes within these criteria, and a qualified nurse or a learner is found guilty of that offence, the police have a duty to report that person to the General Nursing Council. A nurse so reported may then face disciplinary proceedings by the General Nursing Council, the end result of which may be removal from the Register or Roll, or a review of a learner's training.

Civil wrongs are actionable in private law, so proceedings are instituted by the aggrieved person—the plaintiff. The action usually takes the form of the plaintiff serving a High Court writ on the defendant, or a summons being served on the defendant through the County Court. As far as the CPN is concerned, the likely parties to any action are the patient as plaintiff suing the Area Health Authority as employer of the defendant (the nurse involved in the civil wrongs). In civil cases, the outcome results in judgement being given to one party or the other, and this is enforceable through the court against the liable party. The judgement usually involves payment of a sum of money and normally entails bearing the costs of the case.

LEGISLATION AND COMMUNITY PSYCHIATRIC NURSING

Legislation is becoming an increasingly important part of the fabric of English law, a trend which is likely to continue. Clearly there are many Acts of Parliament which impinge directly on the role of the community psychiatric nurse, as a glance at the following list will show:

> Children and Young Persons Act, 1969
> Chronically Sick and Disabled Persons Act, 1970
> Contracts of Employment Act, 1972
> Disabled Persons (Employment) Acts, 1944 and 1958
> Education (Handicapped Children) Act, 1970
> Family Law Reform Act, 1969
> Health and Safety at Work Act, 1974
> Legal Aid and Advice Act, 1949–72

Medicines Act, 1968
Mental Health Act, 1959
Misuse of Drugs Act, 1971
Motor Vehicle (Passenger Insurance) Act, 1971
National Health Service Acts, 1946-77
National Health Service (Injury Benefits) Regulations, 1974
National Insurance (Industrial Injuries) Act, 1965
Nurses Acts—Various
Occupiers Liability Act, 1957
Offences against the Person Act, 1861
Professions Supplementary to Medicine Act, 1960
Social Security Act, 1975
Social Security Benefits Act, 1975
Social Security (Miscellaneous Provisions) Act, 1977
Social Security (Industrial Injuries) (Prescribed Diseases)
    Amendment Regulations, 1977

This is by no means meant to be a comprehensive list, it is simply a sample which occurs to the writer of the legislation which may affect the community psychiatric nurse as a practitioner. It would clearly be quite outside the scope of a chapter like this—which is meant to be but the barest of outlines—to discuss this legislation. We will content ourselves at this stage of development by pointing out the most crucial legislation and making a few comments.

The Mental Health Act, 1959

Whilst a revolutionary piece of legislation in its day, the Mental Health Act, 1959 has fallen into a sad state of disrepair in a number of areas, and is badly in need of a facelift. This should come within the next couple of years and, hopefully, the new Act will cast some light on grey areas of practice in respect of both restraint and treatment. Additionally, it is to be hoped that the move to community care which was prompted by the 1959 Act will be re-emphasised and given the further impetus it merits.

The Mental Health Act, 1959 has been amended by subsequent legislation, as Edwards[4] notes, viz:

The Health Services and Public Health Act, 1968
The Local Authority Social Services Act, 1970
The Local Government Act, 1972
The National Health Services Reorganisation Act, 1973

It is still in need of a basic overhaul, however, in respect of a number of its basic provisions, as Gostin[2] has rightly pointed out.

The overhaul of the Act will need to be a delicate balancing act between the civil rights of patients and the problem of more protection for hospital staff. The competing claims of the National Association for Mental Health (MIND) and the British Association of Social Workers (B.A.S.W.) voicing on one side their disquiet about patients' rights, and on the other side the unions, in particular C.O.H.S.E. (cf. their report: *The Management of Violent or Potentially Violent Patients*), voicing concern over more protection for staff, make the compromise a difficult one for the D.H.S.S. and the Home Office. The problem is, of course, that both sides are right. The issue, in the final analysis, will probably only be resolved in the light of a decision reached by the European Court of Human Rights on cases brought before it by MIND.

All one can do is to urge C.P.N.s to keep an eye open for any White Papers, discussion documents, policy statements published, and contribute whenever possible to what promises to be a very lively discussion. It is time we had the views of nurses on record, to augment those of doctors, social workers, voluntary groups, and all sorts of others who from time to time leap into the verbal fray.

Statutory assaults
The relevant Acts of Parliament here are the following:
>The Offences against the Person Act, 1861
>The Children and Young Persons Act, 1933
>The Sexual Offences Act, 1956
>The Mental Health Act, 1959, and
>The various Road Traffic Acts.

Martin(5) provides a useful discussion of this topic if the reader wishes to follow it up.

The area in which the C.P.N. is most likely to be involved is that of violent behaviour by a patient and the problems caused thereby. The D.H.S.S. paper—HC (76) 11—sets forth the problem, and establishes a basis for further discussion. The circular encourages A.H.A.s to 'review arrangements in each hospital—general as well as psychiatric ...' In addition, S.3 of the Criminal Law Act, 1967, has brought a measure of simplicity to the situation. Prior to that the common law rules enshrined in the 'duty of retreat' doctrine were both complex and uncertain. Whilst they may still have some relevance in construction, S.3, as above, poses the question as to what is reasonable in the particular circumstances in question: viz. 'S.3 (1) A person may use such force as is reasonable in the circumstances in the prevention of crime ...' Community psychiatric nurses are vulnerable in this area—as indeed they are in all areas of statutory assault—for reasons already pointed out, and they should therefore ensure that:

1. their particular A.H.A. has got a written review of the problem which takes account of community nurses, and
2. they are familiar with the pertinent provisions thereof.

The press is very partial to anything which smacks of statutory assault—whether violent or sexual—especially by those involved in the care of the mentally ill/handicapped— and it is as well, therefore, to ensure that you are reading the news rather than making it!

Drugs
It is in this area that nurses most often fall foul of the criminal law. Offences tend to fall into two categories:

1. offences involving abuse to a patient, e.g. administration of a 'prescription only' medicine without a prescription;
2. offences where only the nurse is involved, e.g. obtaining drugs with a forged prescription.

The relevant Acts of Parliament are the following:
   The Medicines Act, 1968
   The Misuse of Drugs Act, 1971.
The position has been complicated somewhat by a recent addition to the Medicines Act, viz. Part III, the bulk of which came into operation on February 1st, 1978. This has been further refined by three Statutory Instruments (No. 987 dealing with Prescription Only Medicines, 988 dealing with Pharmacy and General Sale Products, and 989 dealing with the Miscellaneous Provisions). Additionally, we can expect further legislation in due course on 'the safekeeping of medicine products', as provided for by Part III, S. 66 (1) (f) of the Medicines Act.
   Legislation at best only provides minimum requirements and it is up to individual A.H.A.s to offer administrative guidance to C.P.N.s in order that a comprehensive policy can be prepared and adhered to.
   The Community Psychiatric Nurses Association (C.P.N.A.) monitors the situation continuously, and has prepared a paper on this very thorny question for the guidance of practitioners.
   Regarding medicinal products, the following points are worth bearing in mind:

1. Virtually all injectables are 'prescription only medicines' (P.O.M.s); and P.O.M.s may only be supplied to a C.P.N. via a prescription [Part III, S 58 (2) (a)], or, under Article 10 of the Medicines (Prescriptions Only) Order 1977, in accordance with the written directions of a doctor when supplied in the course of the 'business of a hospital'. (The Act defines 'hospital' as a

'clinic, nursing home or similar institution'—this does not include health centres)! It is possible to be exempted from the prescription requirement (cf. the Medicines (Prescription Only) Order, 1977 and the Medicines (Pharmacy and General Sale—Exemption) Order, 1977), but none of these exemptions covers C.P.N.s at the moment, presumably because such exemption has not yet been requested by C.P.N.s! (Interestingly, where some amelioration of the Part III Legislation has been requested, it has been granted. The case in point—where the R.C.N. applied on behalf of occupational health nurses, and obtained relief under Statutory Instrument No. 987 which came into operation on August 11th, 1978). There may well be a lesson here for C.P.N.s.

2. It is assumed under the Act that 'supply of' and 'carriage of' medicinal products are the same thing—in other words, where a C.P.N. has lawfully been supplied with a medicinal product then there is no criminal liability inherent in the carriage of that medicinal product *per se*.

3. a. In practice, therefore, the normal range of 'products' carried by the average C.P.N. are: the anti-psychiatric depot injections; the anti-Parkinsonism injections; the tranquilising agent injections, all of which are P.O.M.s, and must have been supplied in accordance with (1) above.

b. In order to minimise the risk of incurring criminal liability, the following points are worth noting:

(i) only carry a 24-hour supply;

(ii) always carry all products in a locked case, which must be kept under the C.P.N.s personal supervision, or locked away out of sight in the boot of the car;

(iii) have about your person a properly authenticated indentification card stating your right to carry medicinal products;

(iv) encourage patients wherever possible to collect their own prescriptions;

(v) dispose of patients' medicines no longer required by destroying them in the presence of a relative of theirs, and getting a signature to that effect;

(vi) have in readiness some system of operation designed to provide for the removal of products from a confused/suicidal patient, etc. This will involve the written co-operation of the doctor, pharmacist, and nursing administration;

(vii) ensure that a sound system of recording is in operation;

(viii) ensure that a sound system of storage is in operation at the C.P.N. base.

4. Administration of P.O.M.s should present no problem. C.P.N.s are not exempted from the requirement relating to the administration of P.O.M.s, which are: '... no person may adminster an injectable to another unless he is a doctor, dentist, or veterinarian, or *a person acting in accordance with the directions of such a practitioner*.' Presumably doctors would not prescribe medicines unless they wanted the nurses to administer them!

Regarding Pharmacy Sale (P) medicines (i.e. products not listed in either the Medicines (Prescription Only) Order, 1977, or the Medicines (General Sale List) Order, 1977):

1. Exemption from the regulations regarding supply, under Part III, S. 55 (1), although not a personal exemption under S. 52, is had via a prescription or written order from a doctor designating the medicine for a particular patient.
2. There is no restriction on the administration of P. medicines.

Regarding General Sale List products, the remarks made about P. medicines are equally applicable to G.S.L. products.

Regarding controlled drugs, under the Misuse of Drugs Act, 1971, the picture is somewhat different. 'Possession' is dealt with under that Act, and if therefore it were ever comtemplated that a C.P.N. might carry a 'controlled drug' then the Home Office Drugs Branch should be contacted for advice. The C.P.N.A. is currently (August, 1978) doing just that to ascertain what the general position is!

For offences where there is no patient involvement see '"Personal" offences' below.

Assorted thefts, forgeries and frauds

The relevant Acts of Parliament here are the following:

The Forgery Act, 1913
The Theft Act, 1968.

Unfortunately, nurses, from time to time fall foul of the law in these areas.

The more common offences include:
shoplifting;
thefts from patients;
thefts from place of employment;
miscellaneous thefts;
false accounting;
fraudulent travel.

The commission of such statutory offences can bring a nurse to the attention of the statutory body—the General Nursing Council—with possible unfortunate consequences. In any case, all these offences are criminal in nature and not unnaturally therefore carry their own stigma with them.

'Personal' offences

The sort of offences to which I refer here are the following:
> sexual offences not related to the work situation at all;
> drug abuse, usually involving theft of drugs or forgery of prescriptions;
> alcohol abuse related to the work situation.

This item—'personal' criminal offences—is placed at the end of the section of 'Legislation and Community Psychiatric Nursing' because not all the offences are necessarily statutory in nature and may in fact be common law offences, which do constitute the next section.

It is often considered by nurses that what they do in their own private lives is their own business and has nothing to do with the work situation. This is not so—one of the extra duties which all professionals have imposed on themselves is the necessity of behaving in private life as they would in public life. Statutory bodies are invested, amongst other things, with the responsibility of preserving professional standards, and where a particular individual transgresses well-established bounderies of behaviour then he or she runs the risk of being placed 'beyond the pale'.

THE COMMON LAW AND COMMUNITY PSYCHIATRIC NURSING

The discerning reader will have recognised by now that most statutory offences (i.e. those offences involving breach of legislation, usually an Act of Parliament) with which the C.P.N. is likely to be brought into contact are criminal in nature. It is also true to say that most common law offences which the C.P.N. may encounter are of a civil nature.

Communication

The C.P.N. is a member of a team, often working away from the parent institution, and this therefore presents problems so far as communication is concerned. In practice, generally speaking, it will be questions of treatment and follow-up which may prove most important in this sensitive area. But, especially where the C.P.N. is on an 'open-referral system', assessment may also cause problems in so far as putting others in the picture is concerned: until everyone is in the picture and the team has had a chance to discuss the patient's case, it is the person who took the primary referral who is 'carrying the can'. Judgements made, treatment plans carried out, advice given all have their hazards, but these hazards are lessened if they are shared.

There are a number of cases in which nurses have been involved:

Coles v. Reading H.M.C., 1963
Collins v. Herts. C.C., 1967
Watts v. Brent A.H.A., 1976

In all these cases problems might have been avoided by better communication between doctor, nurse and patient.

A comprehensive recording system is, of course, essential to the maintenance of good communication—indeed, communication in a vast bureaucracy such as the National Health Service could not exist without it! So, all aspects of the care process: assessment, planning, treatment and evaluation, should be recorded, along with all the other paraphernalia which is inherent in working in an organisation, and when recorded, should be made available to the members of the care team.

Consent

Very few patients may be treated against their will under the Mental Health Act, 1959, the obvious exceptions being people on treatment orders such as Ss. 26, 60 and 65. Obviously, informal patients cannot be treated against their will. There is now a school of thought which suggests that certain treatments, e.g. E.C.T. should never be administered to anyone—even patients on treatment orders—without prior discussion and the patient's consent! Be that as it may, the position regarding consent is the following:

> Generally speaking there is no doubt that a patient is entitled to know what is the matter with him, what treatment is proposed and what, if any, serious risks may arise out of that treatment. If he does not know, then he has not consented to the treatment, which in turn means that the practitioners involved could be liable for trespass to the person.(6)

['Trespass to the person' is a civil wrong (a tort in fact), which may take the form of either a 'battery' (physical contact with the person of the plaintiff without consent), or an 'assault' (causing plaintiff to apprehend a contact with his person)]. It is essential, therefore, that the C.P.N. ensures that patients are a willing party to their treatment!

Another intentional tort to the person is 'false imprisonment'. This trespass is 'an act of the defendant which directly and intentionally or negligently causes the confinement of the plaintiff within an area delimited by the defendant'.(7) The cause of such action would normally lie with hospital nurses but C.P.N.s should be aware of this area of the law as it might infringe on their area of practice. If you are responsible for detaining a patient—it does not matter where: it could be in his own home—then you may have committed the civil wrong of false imprisonment, unless of course the patient were subject to detention under the Mental Health Act, 1959.

Confidentiality

As a C.P.N. you may often be in possession of sensitive information in respect of a patient's health, family situation, finances, social circumstances, etc, etc. Such information is, of course, privileged, and should not be disclosed to all and sundry. If it is disclosed in an improper manner, the least the patient can do is to complain to the statutory body or to the employers about the nurse's misconduct. (It should not be forgotten that qualified nurses may be removed from the Register or Roll for professional misconduct as well as for criminal offences—and breach of confidentiality certainly comes within the orbit of professional misconduct!) It is not clear in law if a patient can have recourse to the courts in this matter, but

> Hunter v. Mann, 1974

seems to suggest that a patient so wronged may seek a remedy in either contract or tort. So the preservation of confidentiality is crucial not only in its sense of avoiding possible litigation or complaints, but it also helps to maintain the patient's confidence in the practitioner and thus sustain the therapeutic relationship.

Team members, in making statements or writing reports to each other about patients or clients are protected by 'qualified privilege', i.e. no action may lie for statements or reports made in good faith. Qualified privilege is only lost when bad faith enters in, i.e. when the speaker or writer knows a statement or report to be false and damaging. (Incidentally, qualified privilege also extends to references provided they are given in good faith; here, even careless expression if misleading may make the writer liable to negligence:

> Hedley Byrne v. Heller, 1964).

Defamation of character

Where practitioners make statements or reports about patients or clients which are made in bad faith, then they risk becoming liable for defamation of character. Defamation consists of making a false statement about a person which tends 'to lower the plaintiff in the estimation of right-thinking members of society generally':

> Sim v. Stretch, 1936

There are two types of defamation; libel, which is generally written, and slander, which is generally oral; and the statement or report must of course, be made to a third party. Libel is actionable *per se*, i.e. damage to the plaintiff's reputation is implied; slander is not generally actionable without proof of special damage, i.e. actual damage which is not too remote:

> Lynch v. Knight, 1861.

So, if you as a C.P.N. make false statements or reports about a patient or colleague you risk liability for defamation of character; if you make a careless report which misleads, you risk liability in negligence.

Negligence

Negligence is by far and away the most important of all torts. During the last century it became recognised as a separate tort with district principles involved in its construction; however, vestiges of the old common law still remain, in that negligent acts may still form part of other torts, e.g. trespass and nuisance. The landmark case of

Donoghue v. Stevenson, 1932

paved the way for the tremendous expansion of litigation in this field.

The tort of negligence contains three essential elements:

1. duty of care;
2. breach of duty;
3. resulting damage, cf.

Lochgelly Iron and Coal Co. v. M'Mullan, 1934

So, for a patient (plaintiff) to succeed in an action against an Area Health Authority (defendant), it must be shown that the particular practitioner(s) concerned had a duty towards that patient, that there was breach of that duty, and that the patient in consequence suffered some damage.

That practitioners owe a duty to their clients/patients is well established in a long line of cases from:

Strangeways-Lesmere v. Clayton, 1936
Taylor v. Gray, 1937
Morris v. Winsbury-White, 1937
Mahon v. Osborne, 1939
Ybarra v. Spangard, 1944
Urry and another v. Bierer and another, 1955
Smith v. Brighton, H.M.C., 1958
Junor v. McNichol, 1959
Coles v. Reading, H.M.C., 1963
Collins v. Herts. C.C., 1967

There is no clear definition of the apportionment of responsibility of Area Health Authority personnel for negligent acts. This means that all practitioners must exercise due care in carrying out their duties—liability for negligence may be joint or single depending entirely upon the facts of the case.

What is due care? The standard of care is that expected of an ordinary prudent person. It will, of course, depend on the circumstances—every case always turns on its own facts. A practitioner is expected to show the same kind of competence which would normally be expected of his fellow practitioners—and this of course may ordinarily be determined by 'expert witnesses'. This whole question is comprehensively discussed in a Canadian case:

Chasney v. Anderson;

other cases of interest in this area are:

Jones v. Manchester Corporation, 1952
Roe v. Ministry of Health, 1954
Hatcher v. Black, 1954
Bolam v. Friern H.M.C., 1957
Williams v. North Liverpool H.M.C., 1959
Smith v. Leech Braine & Co., 1962
Hamilton v. Hardy, 1976.

What if a practitioner does become liable in negligence? As Knight(8) has pointed out 'the liability of hospital authorities for negligence of their staff has changed over the years'. The case of

Cassidy v. Minister of Health, 1951

provided a summary of the matter per Lord Denning: the employer (now the Area Health Authority) is vicariously liable for the acts of employees (doctors, nurses, ancillary staff, etc). (This, of course, is always subject to the two provisions—basic to vicarious liability—that the employee must

1. commit a legal wrong;
2. commit the legal wrong in the course of his employment.

Unless these two criteria apply, the employer cannot be vicariously liable). So, provided the two latter provisions apply—and the second is important for C.P.N.s since they often work 'flexitime'—then the Area Health Authority will be vicariously liable for any damage occasioned to your patient by your negligent act.

Vicarious liability as precarious liability for the employee
The matter does not end with vicarious liability unfortunately, because of the questions of personal liability, and duty to the employer under the contract of service. Under the former, a nurse as a practitioner could be sued personally or as a joint tortfessor, and under the latter the employer could sue the employee for breach of implied term of contract, viz. to use reasonable care in the performance of one's duties. For instance in

Urry v. Bierer, 1955

the Court found the surgeon and theatre sister equally to blame, and in

Jones v. Manchester Corporation, 1952

damages were assessed as follows: 80 per cent against the hospital authority and 20 per cent against the doctor. In another case

Romford Ice and Cold Storage Co. v. Lister, 1955
it was held that the employer could recover from their employee—a
lorry driver—the full amount of damages paid to the third party. If this
decision were to presage the case of

Lim v. Camden and Islington A.H.A., 1977
then practitioners would need to look out for themselves in terms of
indemnity insurance. In this case, nearly a quarter of a million pounds
was awarded to the plaintiff—a Malaysian psychiatrist who entered
the Elizabeth Garrett Anderson hospital for a minor gynaecological
operation, and suffered a cardiac arrest which permanently incapaci-
tated her and reduced her to a helpless invalid who would require to be
nursed for the rest of her life. (cf. The Times, December 8th, 1977). In
arriving at the amount of damages to be awarded against the Area
Health Authority, the court took into consideration the question of
inflation—the award was exclusive of both interest and costs. The
Area Health Authority naturally appealed, but whatever the outcome
they would certainly be stuck with a large bill. Cases such as this lead
one to suspect that the day will soon dawn when funds may cease to
become available centrally to meet these huge payments, and Area
Health Authorities may be forced to think in terms of redress against
their employees. It is imperative, therefore, that C.P.N.s—and for that
matter all nurses—have some sort of personal indemnity insurance.
The C.P.N.A. is still looking into this question, and it becomes ever
more important as time goes by. Indemnity insurance is generally
available in three ways:

1. through a professional body;
2. through a union;
3. through an insurance broker in respect of a private indemnity
   insurance policy.

It is worth bearing in mind that employers are vicariously liable not
just for negligent acts of employees, but for any tortious act; and whilst
negligence is by far and away the most dangerous tort for the C.P.N. it
is, as has been shown above, not the only one the nurse may fall foul of
by any means. So make sure you are covered, and whilst doing so
remember to look at the question of costs also—the damages awarded
in the Lim case did *not* include costs, and of course they can be extremely heavy. Normally the party becoming liable for damages has
the costs also awarded against him, and if your indemnity insurance
policy does not provide for costs (both yours and the other party's)
then it is clearly less than satisfactory.

If you, as a C.P.N., are not covered by a suitable indemnity
insurance policy giving you protection against personal liability, and if

your employers seek redress against you because they become vicariously liable for damages on your behalf, then you may find yourself paying off a debt that you cannot get to the end of—for example, the court may order one third of your salary to be paid in liquidation of the debt until it is cleared, if it ever is!

This whole area of the law is very unsatisfactory at the present time. New Zealand has tackled the problem by introducing a scheme of 'no-fault compensation'—an automatic right of compensation upon injury. A recent Royal Commission rejected such a solution in this country. The writer believes that while the present system continues, one solution would be for nurses to have indemnity insurance as a term of contract in the same way that newly-qualified doctors are obliged to join a defence organisation. I'm sure that it is not beyond the wit of Area Health Authorities to organise something suitable—in the final analysis everyone would be better off—patient, practitioner and employer!

THE C.P.N. IN COURT
Normally, a nurse is likely to appear in court as:

1. a defendant in either a criminal case or a civil action;
2. a witness in order to give evidence as a result of professional involvement—again the case might be either criminal or civil.

The only advice one can offer to a nurse being proceeded against is to seek competent legal advice at the earliest possible moment. Members of professional bodies and unions can avail themselves, usually freely, of legal advice from the relevant departments. Those who are not members of such associations should see their solicitor. To be on the wrong end of either a criminal or civil case can be very costly, so any money spent in forestalling that eventuality is money extremely well spent! Your advisors will tell you of all your duties, responsibilities and rights, including legal aid.

Nurses, particularly community nurses, are sometimes called upon to appear in court as witnesses. I can do no better than refer practitioners who are so called upon to the D.H.S.S. Health Services Management document dated January, 1976, where the position of the nurse is discussed (cf. HS1 B(1) January, 1976).

STATEMENTS
Nurses may be called upon to make statement from time to time. Statements may be requested by:

1. the employer;
2. the police;

3. the courts;
4. the coroner.

It goes without saying that the greatest care must be exercised in the writing of a statement. Mistakes or careless language which tends to mislead could have grave consequences both personally and professionally. It need hardly be said either that the truth must be meticulously adhered to at all times.

The following points may be worth noting about the making of statements:

1. If the statement is to be made about a living person, the patient's permission should first of all be obtained if the circumstances allow.
2. The police are not entitled to demand information, except under a few statutory circumstances, e.g. under the Road Traffic Acts, under the provisions of S. 5 of the Criminal Law Act, 1967 (cf. Speller.(9)). Although there is in general no legal duty to give information to the police, there may be a public or social duty to do so: it may well be a matter of conscience!
3. The courts or a judge in chambers are entitled to demand information. You and/or your records can be compelled *subpoena* to appear in court; failure to comply, is 'contempt of court' and a criminal offence.
4. In general, the content of a written statement might be somewhat as follows:
   a. the statement should be dated at the top;
   b. there should be a preamble stating to whom and for what purpose the statement is being made;
   c. the introduction should provide the basic statistics on the subject: name, address, etc., etc;
   d. the main body of the statement should concern itself with a factual account of the case/incident, etc., etc., giving all the necessary details in chronological order;
   e. the next paragraph should provide, if appropriate, an account of the matter by others, e.g. the subject, witnesses, etc., etc;
   f. finally, one might conclude by summarising the facts. If one is in the position of being an 'expert witness', opinions may be expressed, but:
      (i) they must be supported by the facts, and
      (ii) the facts must be clearly understood by the court, with technical terms explained, etc.

Even so, the witness may be required to give oral evidence at the instance of either party. If you pass an opinion you must make it quite plain that you are so doing by prefacing your remarks by some such phrase as:

> In my opinion ...
> In my view ...
> I believe that ...
> It would seem to me that ...
> It is apparent that ...
> I think that ...

g. the statement must be signed at the bottom of each page by the person making it.

5. In criminal proceedings, Ss. 2 and 8 of the Criminal Justice Act, 1967, and the Magistrates Court Act, 1967, allow for written statements to be used in proceedings, provided the statement complies with certain prescribed conditions:
a. the statement must be signed by the person making it;
b. copies of the statement must be served on the parties to the proceedings;
c. none of the parties to the proceedings must object to the statement being tendered as evidence in court—parties have seven days from service of the statement during which to object;
d. the statement must end with the words:

> This statement, consisting of X pages, each signed by me, is true to the best of my knowledge and belief and I make it knowing that if it is tendered in evidence, I shall be liable to prosecution if I have knowingly stated in it anything which I know to be false or do not believe to be true.
>
> (Criminal Justice Act, 1967).

False statements made wilfully, amount to perjury (Perjury Act, 1911 via S. 89 of the Criminal Justice Act, 1967). (Interestingly enough, although there is, in general, no compulsion to give information to the police, where one does it could be an offence to give false or misleading information. cf.
Rice v. Connolly, 1966).
If a statement contains anything of a 'hearsay' nature the rules of evidence normally relating to this apply.

6. Documentary evidence is also admissible in court, and indeed may be demanded via a '*subpoena duces tecum*', i.e. the witness is required to come to the court with the particular document. (Documents can be produced to the court on their own also). So nursing records of whatever kind could be sent for by a court—which serves to emphasise what has been said above, viz. the importance of keeping accurate and factual records. Whilst such records are indeed subject to qualified privilege and therefore not liable to an action for defamation of character, it is

also true to say that poor records will leave a poor impression of those who made them.

7. On a point of interest:
   a. Re: Burden of proof:
   the evidential burden always rests on the complaining party, whether that be a prosecutor or plaintiff;
   b. Re: Standard of proof:
   in criminal cases the prosecutor must prove the charge against the accused 'beyond all reasonable doubt'—R. v. White, 1865;
   in civil actions the plaintiff must show cause 'on the balance of probability'—Cooper v. Slade, 1858.

ADVICE TO PATIENTS

Nurses who work in the community clearly have far greater contact with the patient in society as it were, and will therefore get to know the patient's domestic, family, financial and social circumstances quite well in many cases. This being so, the C.P.N. may well find himself being asked for advice of a legal or quasi-legal nature on a whole range of topics as they affect the rights of mental/mental handicap patients—topics such as:

> guardianship;
> mental health review tribunals;
> The Court of Protection;
> contracts in general;
> marriage;
> divorce;
> children;
> wills;
> the right to vote;
> jury service;
> banks;
> insurance;
> allowances

may well crop up, plus many others. Whilst one cannot expect a C.P.N. to be a walking encyclopaedia of legal knowledge, a working knowledge nevertheless would be more than useful. It is clearly outside the scope of a chapter such as this—which is only meant to be a mere outline—to cover such topics. The nurse who wishes to acquire such knowledge, however, will find it in an excellent little book: '*A Guide to the Law Affecting Mental Patients.*' (10)

THE EXTENSION OF THE NURSE'S ROLE

The role of the nurse has undoubtedly been extended considerably during recent years. One can think of a number of areas in which this is so:

1. in A & E—minor suturing, endotracheal intubation, vaccination
2. in anaesthetics—I/V therapy, care of sophisticated hardware
3. behaviour therapy/modification
4. client-centred therapy
5. intensive therapy in coronary care and head injuries—I/V therapy, care of sophisticated machinery
6. medicine, e.g. the stoma care nurse
7. patient assessment
8. prescribing, e.g. the oral contraceptive pill
9. in haematology and renal dialysis—I/V therapy and care of sophisticated machinery
10. the psychotherapies
11. in the operating theatre
12. vaccination/immunisation generally
13. venepuncture—carried out in a number of areas.

There may well be other areas which don't occur to the writer. The nursing press has carried much on the topic, and the D.H.S.S. has not been lacking either:

CMO (76) 9 CNO (76)11, May 24th, 1976

HC (76) 26

HC (77) 22

'Medical manpower—the next twenty years,' 1978.

The problem is not just a professional one, it is very much a legal one also. Broadly speaking, the situation is that most if not all of the techniques involved in the recent extension of the nurse's role referred to above fall outside the role of the nurse as circumscribed by custom and practice.

The traditional role of the nurse, however, is rapidly changing and therefore expanding beyond the confines of custom and practice. In order to come to terms with this ever-altering situation, some mechanism must be devised which allows for the resolution of the question of professional boundaries whilst at the same time maintaining maximum service flexibility in the interests of the patient. Such a mechanism demands that the person who by tradition performed such and such a function, e.g. I/V therapy, should delegate said function to another person who is willing to take it on. This, of course, calls for the voluntary co-operation of both parties. Such co-operation will probably depend on the attitude of the employer—the Area Health Authority—as expressed through its policy for dealing with this particular problem. Doctors, for instance, would probably be less than keen to delegate responsibility to nurses who had not had specialised training—this is where the J.B.C.N.S. courses are of great importance! Nurses on the other hand might well feel that in addition to post-basic training in a particular area (or in-service training as a second best), they would also like to be comforted in the knowledge that should they make a mistake and thereby be guilty of a negligent act then the Area Health Authority would not only be vicariously liable on their behalf but also would not subsequently proceed against them in the courts for redress.

To summarise then:

1. All parties, viz. the Area Health Authority, the doctor, and the nurse must agree to the particular delegated duty.
2. This agreement should be formalised in writing via an 'instrument of delegation'.
3. The nurse should be specially trained in the use of the technique/machine, etc. This is best done via a J.B.C.N.S. course where such exists. (In-service training is a poor substitute).
4. The Area Health Authority should make clear to all concerned its policy on vicarious liability in the area of delegated responsibility, bearing in mind that the nurse making the mistake is the negligent party if the duty has been properly delegated.

The role of the mental nurse has been considerably extended as may be seen from the above list (the role of the mental handicap nurse lesser so perhaps). C.P.N.s are in a position, as has been mentioned many times throughout this book, to become fully-fledged practitioners in the proper sense of the term. The absorption of specialisms such as behaviour therapy/modification, client-centred therapy, crisis-intervention work, patient assessment and the psychotherapies into the generalist role of the C.P.N. does not call for the same sort of formal delegation that is necessary for general nurses, because the doctor cannot lay claim, in the area of mental illness/handicap, to the sole exercise of these functions by custom and practice. Such a claim would indubitably be hotly disputed by analysts, psychologists and social workers to name but a few! So the crucial factor for C.P.N.s is training, and then more training!

The authors of this book are extremely keen to see all nurses extend their role; they feel that mental/mental handicap nurses are as a group best placed to do so! The writer of this chapter is however particularly keen to see that nurses extend their role only where appropriate safeguards exist!

REFERENCES

1. Szasz, T. S. (1974) *Law, Liberty and Psychiatry*. London: Routledge & Kegan Paul Ltd.
2. Gostin, L. O. (1975 and 1977) *A Human Condition*. Vols. 1 and 2. MIND (National Association for Mental Health), London.
3. Williams, G. (1969) *Learning the Law*. 8th edn. London: Stevens & Sons.
4. Edwards, A. H. (1975) *Mental Health Services*. London: Shaw & Sons Ltd.
5. Martin, C. R. A. (1973) *Law relating to Medical Practice*. London: Pitman Medical.
6. Whincup, M. H. (1978) *Legal Aspects of Medical and Nursing Service*. Beckenham: Ravenswood Publications Ltd.
7. Street, H. (1968) *The Law of Torts*. 4th edn. London: Butterworths.
8. Knight, B. (1976) *Legal Aspects of Medical Practice*. 2nd edn. Edinburgh: Churchill Livingstone.
9. Speller, S. R. (1971) *Law Relating to Hospitals and Kindred Institutions*. 5th. edn. London: H. K. Lewis & Co. Ltd.
10. Venables, H. D. (1975) *A Guide to the Law Affecting Mental Patients*. London: Butterworths.

FURTHER READING

Farndale, W. A. J. (1976) *Medical Negligence*. Beckenham: Ravenswood Publications Ltd.
Farndale, W. A. J. and Larman, E. C. (1976) *Legal Liability for Claims Arising from Hospital Treatment*. Beckenham: Ravenswood Publications Ltd.

TABLE OF STATUTES

Offences against the Person Act, 1861.
Perjury Act, 1911.
Forgery Act, 1913.
Nurses' Act, 1919—present.
Road Traffic Acts, 1930—present.
Children and Young Persons' Act, 1933 and 1969.
Disabled Persons (Employment) Acts, 1944 and 1958.
National Health Service Acts, 1946–77.
Sexual Offences Act, 1956.
Occupiers' Liability Act, 1957.
Mental Health Act, 1959.
Professions supplementary to Medicine Act, 1960.
National Insurance (Industrial Injuries) Act, 1965.
Criminal Justice Act, 1967.
Criminal Law Act, 1967.
Magistrates' Courts' Act, 1967.
Theft Act, 1968.
Medicines Act, 1968.
Health Services and Public Health Act, 1968.
Chronically Sick and Disabled Persons Act, 1970.
Education (Handicapped Children) Act, 1970.
Local Authority Social Service Act, 1970.
Legal Aid and Advice Act, 1971.
Misuse of Drugs Act, 1971.

Motor Vehicle (Passenger Insurance) Act, 1971.
Contracts of Employment Act, 1972.
European Communities Act, 1972.
Local Government Act, 1972.
N.H.S. Reorganisation Act, 1973.
Health and Safety of Work Act, 1974.
Social Security Act, 1975.
Social Security Benefits Act, 1975.
Social Security (Miscellaneous Provisions) Act, 1977.

N.B. Not all of these Acts are referred to directly in the text, but they are included in case the reader requires a point of reference.

INDEX OF INSTRUMENTS

National Health Service (Injury Benefits) Regulations, 1974.
Social Security (Industrial Injuries) (Prescribed Diseases) Amendment Regulations, 1977.
Medicines (Prescription Only) Order, 1977.
Medicines (Pharmacy and General Sale—Exemption) Order, 1977.
Medicines (General Sale List) Order, 1977.
Medicines (Prescription Only) Amendment (No. 2) Order, 1978.
Medicines (Pharmacy and General Sale—Exemption) Amendment Order, 1978.
Medicines (Sale or Supply) (Miscellaneous Provisions) Amendment Regulations, 1978.

LIST OF CASES

Bolam v. Friern H.M.C., [**1957**] 2 All E.R. 18.
Burbury v. Jackson, [1917] 1 K.B. 16.
Cassidy v. Minister of Health, [1951] 1 All E.R. 574.
Chasney v. Anderson, [1950] 4 D.L.R. 223.
Coles v. Reading H.M.C. (1963), Times, Jan. 3rd.
Collins v. Herts C.C., [1947] 1 All E.R. 633.
Cooper v. Slade (1858), 1 H.L.C. 746.
Donoghue v. Stevenson, [1932] A.C. 562.
Hamilton v. Hardy (1976), 549 P.2d. 1099.
Hatcher v. Black and Others, [1954] Times, Jul. 2nd.
Hedley Byrne v. Heller, [1964] A.C. 465.
Hunter v. Mann (1974), Times, Feb. 9th.
Jones v. Manchester Corporation, [1952] 1 All E.R. 125.
Junor v. McNichol (1959), Times, Mar. 26th.
Lim v. Camden and Islington Area Health Authority (1977), Times, Dec. 8th.
Lochgelly Iron and Coal Co. v. M'Mullan, [1934] A.C.1.
Lynch v. Knight (1861), 9 H.L.Cas. 577.
Mahon v. Osborne, [1939] 1 All E.R. 535.
Morris v. Winsbury-White, [1937] 4 All E.R. 494.
R. v. White (1865), 4 F. & F. 383.
Rice v. Connolly, [1966] 2 Q.B. 414.
Roe v. Minister of Health and Others, [1954] 2 Q.B. 66
Romford Ice and Cold Storage Co. Ltd., v. Lister, [1955] 2 W.L.R. 158.
Sim v. Stretch, [1936] 2 All E.R. 1237.
Smith v. Brighton H.M.C. (1958), Times, May 2nd.
Smith v. Leech Braine & Co. Ltd., [1962] 2 Q.B. 405.
Strangeways-Lesmere v. Clayton, [1936] 1 All E.R. 484.
Taylor v. Gray, [1937] 4 D.L.R. 123.
Urry and Another v. Bierer and Another, [1955] Times, July 15th.

Watts v. Brent Area Health Authority (1976), London Evening News, Feb. 5th.
Williams v. North Liverpool H.M.C. (1959), Times, Jan. 17th.
Ybarra v. Spangard (1944), 154 Pac. 2d. 687 (Cal).

9

Key areas in community psychiatric nursing development

Community psychiatric nursing has been developing for a number of years now, more quickly in some areas, often due to foresight and finance, and much more comprehensively in psychiatry than in mental handicap. Despite its meteoric rise, it is already showing signs of maturity—its star is definitely in the ascendant!

Progress has been achieved through a variety of approaches, and much imagination has been displayed in the establishment of the present network of services. There is always a danger, of course, that institutionalisation may set in and this must be prevented at all costs.

The signs are already there that this can be done—training courses exist, research, both large-scale and small-scale, has been carried out and a professional association founded.

These three variables—education, research and professional organisation—must be considered as key areas in the development of community psychiatric nursing, and a short discussion of each, therefore, now follows.

SECTION A

Education

The present situation is that the course leading to the Community Psychiatric Nursing Certificate is controlled and validated by the Joint Board of Clinical Nursing Studies. This body controls the syllabuses of the clinical nursing courses for nurses after registration or enrolment covering a wide range of specialisms from renal, onco-logical, and intensive care nursing to behaviour modification, advanced psychiatry and course 800, community psychiatric nursing. The present course consists of a basic community psychiatric nursing course with a mental handicap option. The format of the course is as follows: 16 weeks at a Polytechnic and 23 weeks' field work consisting of two contrasting placements with community psychiatric nursing teams and a short placement in primary health care. The final 12 weeks are spent on supervised practice with the seconding authority during which time case-studies and/or a piece of research is undertaken. The syllabus covers such topics as psychology, sociology, law, health education, social administration as well as the principles and practice of community psychiatric nursing and the specialised therapies. Active consideration is at present being given to a re-structuring of the syllabus. The present system of a basic course with a mental handicap option is unsatisfactory, particularly for nurses specialising in this field. Whilst much of the course content relates to both fields of nursing, a different orientation is required for each. It would thus be preferable to have a common core of subject matter which is then related to the particular branch of the service by means of tutorials or seminars, and two self-contained options or modules for psychiatric and mental handicap nursing. Such a syllabus is expected to be issued by the J.B.C.N.S. in the near future.

Whilst this change is eminently desirable and welcomed, the other change currently being undertaken, namely courses based on hospitals rather than a centre of higher education, is more questionable and may not be in the best interests of the developing profession or indeed the client. The polytechnic-based courses have easy access to eminent academics, researchers, and practitioners as well as a wide range of field work placements. The higher education establishment has a far wider selection of journals, books and reference material on its shelves than a nurse education department in a hospital could hope to have available, and has access through inter-library loan to almost any printed material published anywhere.

A danger of regional courses is that they will become parochial and insular, thereby not benefitting from the experience to be gained from the very different services operating in other geographical areas. This will not encourage diversification, or the introduction of new ideas and will thus result in stagnation. Any large-scale development of regional courses will counter the momentum of this exciting branch of psychiatric nursing and will result in the excellent progress so far achieved coming to an untimely halt.

The current situation with the polytechnic-based courses is that, as a result of inadequate basic training, more time than is warranted is being taken up filling the fundamental gaps of basic training, overcoming the overriding commitment to the 'medical model' of care, and re-orientating the nurse to a more client-centred, less institutional approach to patient care.

As liberal progressive thinking percolates slowly through the training schemes leading to State Registration, it should be less necessary to spend time on models of care, the nursing progress (except as it applies to community nursing) current developments in psychiatry and mental handicap. Rather more time could then be devoted towards the dynamics of family life, family therapy, social and cultural factors in relation to mental disorder, the extension of the nurses role, an examination of alternative strategies·for care and the development of a truly community based, community orientated service. The nurse could then become a professional consultant on nursing and community care, making nursing decisions, executing nursing treatments without reference to other professionals or agencies, although keeping such personnel as is necessary duly informed.

The advent of the 'Briggs Report' will make higher educational certificates in specialised branches of nursing all the more important. 'Generic Jenny'—the social worker has not been shown to be the great success it was anticipated. This lesson must not be overlooked when considering the future of nurse education. The community service will need to develop specialised nurses within the teams if the needs of clients are to be adequately met. It is not possible for all nurses to be good practitioners with all clients. A degree of specialisation will be required in such areas as child and adolescent psychiatry, primary prevention, psycho-sexual counselling, alcoholism or the growing problem of psycho geriatrics. These and other specialised areas will require the development of specialised courses perhaps under the auspices of the J.B.C.N.S. However, as the basic training improves, a modular course catering for specialisms within the basic community nursing course structure should be possible. In the field·of mental handicap the future is less certain. The National Development Group advocate mental handicap community teams, the Court Report (*Fit for the Future*) advocates community handicap teams for children necessitating the specialised training of health visitors. The 'Peggy Jay' Report relating to the future of nurse training for the mentally handicapped, imminent and eagerly awaited may make fundamental changes to basic and post-basic training with a possible major change in philosophy. The training, and control of the service may be vested in the social service departments rather than the health authorities as at present. Better education and a degree of specialisation will still be essential.

The care of the mentally disordered in the community requires nurse practitioners who are well trained, well educated with a breadth of sound knowledge, skills and expertise. The nurse should then be in a position to initiate change, have insight into problems and their solution, operate independently of bureaucratic structures, yet be sufficiently politically aware, and able to develop and sustain an argument to ensure the best service for their clients. To this end it is important to select people of sufficient calibre that they are able to cope with advanced study. The courses should be well-balanced, intellectually stimulating, designed to encourage creative thinking and a questioning, problem-solving approach. The course should not only equip the nurse to practice, but also to be able to adapt the service to meet the changing needs and maintain the progress to professionalism and professional recognition.

SECTION B

Research

No vocational discipline, such as community psychiatric nursing, which has a high clinical content, can hope to advance without a comprehensive research base. Good nursing practice must rely on a sound theoretical infrastructure—the nurse's role in relation to function, attitudes and skills must initially be described and then, hopefully, compared and evaluated. Similarly, the multiplicity of criteria involved in patient care, teamwork, the structure and operation of services, specialisms within the general field of community psychiatric nursing, and many other areas must be isolated, explored and brought into the body of knowledge which needs to be built up in relation to community psychiatric nursing. Theory and practice must be kept in step if the discipline is to advance along the right lines.

Research into mental nursing has been sporadic to say the least. Taking the last war as a starting point (there is little use in looking further than that because one would not see anything), the following are among the projects of note:

1. Goddard, H. A.(1) (on behalf of the Manchester Regional Hospital Board and the University of Manchester) undertook between 1952 and 1954 an analysis of the work of mental nurses with a view to utilising a scarce resource in the best possible way. The team he led looked at both a mental hospital and a mental deficiency hospital (the terms current in those days!). The tool they used was job analysis based on observation. They looked at a number of issues related mainly to formation, and were able to arrive at twenty-two conclusions —most of them to do with:

   a. the character and scope of the work of the ward staff;
   b. the redeployment of the present staff;
   c. the recruitment of additional staff;
   d. a reconsideration of the training and role of the mental nurse.

   2 A Liverpool University(2) study conducted by their Department

of Social Science, took the nature of a survey of two hospitals. Much smaller in scope than the Manchester study (the report covered only some six pages), observations were made under a number of headings mostly to do with shortage and recruitment problems. Despite its brevity the report contains many useful and visionary comments.

3. Another 'job analysis' kind of study was carried out again around the same time, this time by Oppenheim(3). It was conducted in a training hospital in the United Kingdom and the three main findings were as follows:

a. student nurses spent far too much time on domestic work during which there was no real contact with the patient;

b. no strict selection system was in use regarding student nurses;

c. attitude and motivation of the nurses towards their training was unsatisfactory—perceived their role as domestic rather than therapeutic or supportive.

4. John, A. L.(4) carried out a study of the psychiatric nurse a few years later—in the late fifties. She used four hospitals, and carried out a descriptive survey involving the use of four separate but complementary methods: questionnaire, diaries kept by student staff, participant observation, and interviews of a random sample of all grades of nursing staff. She presented her findings under ten headings as follows:

a. the working situation;

b. type of patient;

c. type of nurse;

d. type of work;

e. working conditions;

f. communications;

g. recruitment, selection and training;

h. health;

i. length of service;

j. morale and efficiency.

Her conclusions were rather gloomy, but then, things *were* rather gloomy!

5. It was over ten years later that the next significant study took place, that of Altschul(5) at the Royal Edinburgh Hospital. She looked at patient–nurse interaction patterns in a number of acute psychiatric wards. She made use of observations and interviews, and was able to indicate a relationship between a number of variables, e.g. age, sex, class and the frequency and duration of interactions.

6. Towell, D.(6) working at a psychiatric hospital in the early seventies and using participant observation, demonstrated that nurses' perceptions of their function were shaped by the work setting; and that in fact role involves a cluster of potential performances each one of

which may be cued in by a different scene setting. (This study in some ways reinforced the findings of Caine and Smail in a previous study, 1967–8(7)).

7. The D.H.S.S. Research Fellowship Scheme has occasioned a number of studies being carried out in the field, most of which are, as yet, unpublished. They include the work of Carr(8), already referred to elsewhere, on the D.G.H. psychiatric unit.

As can be seen from this very brief resumé, we are not exactly overdone with research in the field of mental health/handicap, albeit that there are studies other than those mentioned. The field of community psychiatric nursing is even more lacking in this respect, there being just two major studies:

1. Sladden(9) carried out a descriptive study of one Community Psychiatric Nursing Service based at a psychiatric teaching hospital in Edinburgh. She concentrated on nurse–patient contact and the process and content of nurse–patient interaction. Her main finding was that the service operated only as an after-care agency by and large, and that this was very much in the context of the hospital.

2. Parnell, J. W.(10) carried out a broad descriptive study to determine differences in approach to the organisation of community psychiatric nursing.

We at Manchester Polytechnic are very keen to see C.P.N.s involved in small-scale research projects. There is a danger—and one has seen some evidence—of research becoming institutionalised and thus controlled. This is abhorrent to the enquiring mind, and must be counteracted at all costs: one way of achieving this is through small-scale research, i.e. research aimed at solving some local problem and fulfilling some local need, etc. Our students are encouraged to engage in this kind of research, and we have been able to institute a 'Manchester Polytechnic Community Psychiatric Nursing Research Monograph Series' based on our students' efforts entirely. A number of community psychiatric services are already in existence as a result of students' projects, and often running along the lines suggested in the research project. Students have also carried out regional and national surveys. It may perhaps come as a sobering thought to those stout pillars of the research establishment, and to those who support them, that while their weighty tomes are bending some library shelf somewhere undisturbed except by half an inch of dust, the rather slimmer fruits of small-scale research are actually helping to make the wheels go round!

SECTION C

Unions and professional organisations and community psychiatric nurses

The establishment of any new type of nursing service will mean that they will have special needs and requirements in the way of professional representation and support. Community psychiatric nurses are not exempt from these needs and a number of developments have taken place in this area. The Confederation of Health Service Employees, National Union of Public Employees and the Royal College of Nursing have all made token gestures towards the support and requirements of community psychiatric nurses. But with little knowledge of the specialist needs involved, they served only to emphasise the vacuum in this area which the C.P.N.A. eventually came along and filled.

The Community Psychiatric Nurses' Association (C.P.N.A.) was founded initially as a regional association for community psychiatric nurses in the north west of England and went under the title of The North West Community Psychiatric Group. The inaugural meeting took place in Bolton on Tuesday, September 3rd, 1974, and was attended by community psychiatric nurses from the north west and Merseyside regions. The purpose of this meeting was to create a forum for the discussion of all matters relating to community psychiatric nurses.

Arising out of this first meeting a working party set up to consider the formation of the group and eight months later, on Thursday May 29th, 1975, at a meeting held in a Manchester hotel, it was suggested that the group become an association. To that end, a formal committee was elected and regular meetings decided on. The first meeting of the North West Community Psychiatric Nurses' Association was held at Winwick Hospital on Tuesday June 24th, 1975. Thus began the formation of a professional group with a distinct identity—a group capable of looking after the specific interests of community psychiatric nurses.

It soon became apparent to the association that it was too parochial in its outlook and with that in mind the prefix 'North West' was dropped from the title, which thus became the Community Psychiatric Nurses' Association (C.P.N.A.).

In the meetings that followed during the latter part of 1975 objectives and a structure were developed for the C.P.N.A. These were embodied in a formal constitution which was submitted to the Charity Commissions in November, 1975. The constitution was accepted on its first reading and the Community Psychiatric Nurses'

Association became a registered charity in April, 1976. (No. 271008).

The objectives of the C.P.N.A. as embodied in the constitution are as follows:

1. To promote the art and science of psychiatric nursing in the community;
2. To further the education and training of community psychiatric nurses and help monitor their professional standards;
3. To act as a representative body for community psychiatric nurses;
4. To provide a means of communication between members of the Association.

Meanwhile, in the south of England, community psychiatric nurses were coming together and beginning to talk about the need for a representative body. A meeting planned for community psychiatric nurses in the Wessex Region and to be held at Park Prewitt Hospital on June 18th, 1976 served as a focus for all this activity and found itself acting as host to community psychiatric nurses from all over the south of England.

The steering committee set up as a result of this meeting was invited by the C.P.N.A. to a meeting at Winwick Hospital during September, 1976, and a small representative group made the journey to Warrington. As a result of that meeting the steering committee decided to recommend to community psychiatric nurses throughout the south that the two bodies unite.

One other body which has shown a marked interest in community psychiatric nurses has been the Queen's Nursing Institute. Parnell(10) has undertaken a detailed study looking at psychiatric nursing in the community. This was undertaken as a Ph.D. study while research officer at the Queen's Institute.

Parnell's study is probably the most detailed look at community psychiatric nursing that has been undertaken to date. The study was undertaken 'to obtain information on the current and future development of psychiatric nursing in the community'.

The study goes into considerable detail about the professional background and preparation of staff involved, the operation of the services and the day to day work involvement. Views were also sought from staff about the current and future development of community psychiatric nursing. The study has obvious hallmarks of general nursing influence with some questioning based on the medical model approach but as a piece of work will doubtless be influential in the future development of community psychiatric nursing. Although the interest of any body of people in community psychiatric nursing is welcome, the influences of such bodies inexperienced in psychiatric nursing need to be be examined carefully.

This is no doubt that the community psychiatric nursing fraternity is still a small voice in a large gathering of other nursing services but the establishment of its own professional organisation can do nothing but good towards the development and consolidation of its own needs and interests.

REFERENCES

1. Goodard, H. A. (1955) *The Work of the Mental Nurse.* Manchester: Manchester University Press.
2. The University of Liverpool (1954) *The Work and Status of Mental Nurses.* Liverpool: Liverpool University Pamphlet.
3. Oppenheim, A. M. (1954) *The Function and Training of Mental Nurses.* London: Chapman and Hall Ltd.
4. John, A. L. (1961) *A Study of the Psychiatric Nurse.* Edinburgh: E. & S. Livingstone Ltd.
5. Altschul, A. (1972) *Patient–Nurse Interaction.* Edinburgh: Churchill Livingstone.
6. Towell, D. (1975) *Understanding Psychiatric Nursing.* London: Royal College of Nursing.
7. Caine, T. and Smail, D. (1969) *The Treatment of Mental Illness.* London: University of London Press.
8. Carr, P. J. (1979) 'To describe the role of the nurse working in a psychiatric unit which is situated in a district general hospital complex.' Unpublished Ph.D. Thesis, University of Manchester.
9. Sladden, S. (1979) *Psychiatric Nursing in the Community.* Edinburgh: Churchill Livingstone. (To be published).
10. Parnell, J. W. (1977) 'Psychiatric Nursing in the community.' Unpublished Ph.D. Thesis, University of Surrey.

10

A blueprint for the future

We suggested at the end of the first chapter of this book that a new era is about to dawn for mental and mental handicap nurses. Shakespeare said:

All the world's a stage,
And all the men and women merely players:
They have their exits and their entrances.

(As You Like It, II, vii.)

Community psychiatric nursing has just made its entrance onto the health stage, and seems set to play an important part in that arena during what remains of this millenium and beyond.

Practitioners working in this field are being afforded the opportunity—never given before the mental and mental handicap nurses—of creating for their respective professions a role which is at one and the same time independent (in the sense of practitioner status) and interdependent (in the sense of the teamwork approach). In this way will community psychiatric nurses be enabled to deliver care to their patients, which is both singular (in the sense that it is based on the unique contribution which mental and mental handicap nurses are able to make because of their training, experience and high level of patient contact) and comprehensive (in the sense that it benefits fully from the teamwork approach). Many mistakes have been made along the path of professional development—perhaps now is the time to start putting them right!

Having read the chapters intervening between the first and last you will no doubt have your own ideas as to how the future of community psychiatric nursing will shape up. We are going to suggest a few ideas of our own which we think merit consideration when pondering where we go from her. (They are not necessarily in any particular order.)

PSYCHIATRIC NURSES IN THE COMMUNITY

1. Community psychiatric nurses have needed to be generalists to begin with—and that is the way their training will continue—but it

may well happen that eventually they will specialise, e.g. in psycho-geriatrics, or with children etc. Perhaps the typical community psychiatric nurse of the future will have done three trainings: basic, community psychiatric, plus one specialism, say psychogeriatrics, child and adolescent psychiatry, behaviour therapy, drugs/alcoholism, psychotherapy/counselling, forensic psychiatry, etc.

2. The eventual path of community psychiatric nursing must be in the direction of true 'primary' care and consequently call for greater awareness of and involvement in health education.
3. There will be a tendency for services to become more compre-hensive and therefore more uniform in that they will 'service' both hospital and primary health care team!
4. Community psychiatric nurses may well find that they must be prepared to accept statutory responsibilities if their role is to continue to expand.
5. Community psychiatric nurses will almost certainly be deployed on a 'per population' basis rather than the present unsatisfactory, *ad hoc* arrangements, whereby community psychiatric nurses are not even separately identified in staffing returns to the D.H.S.S. (cf. Community Outlook, August 1978).

MENTAL HANDICAP NURSES IN THE COMMUNITY

1. There will be a progressive dissolution of the historical connection between psychiatry and mental handicap, so that the handicapped will come to be seen as disadvantaged rather than diseased.
2. The nurse will become an equal member of the community mental handicap team, and will be recognised as a specialist in their own right. There will in turn therefore be less concern about professional —and geographical—boundaries.
3. There will be an increasing emphasis on neighbourhood resources through which people will be encouraged to care for the disabled in their own community—the caring community.
4. We shall see the development of a comprehensive community nursing service, based on clients' needs and utilising a systematic care plan.
5. The district handicap team will be developed to cater for all handicaps of all ages. This will mean specialisation—but the specialisation should be grounded in terms of the effects of the handicap rather than its cause.

GENERAL POINTS FOR COMMUNITY PSYCHIATRIC NURSES

1. It will be necessary to be much more politically—and legally (the

two often go together)—aware than in the past. All the goodwill in the world will achieve nothing unless the wheels are set in motion: knowing how to do this, and doing it will be essential if progress is to be maintained.

2. The behavioural perspective must be kept firmly in view.

3. Research is essential to the maintenance of good practice—the more the field expands, the more will research become necessary. The academic process—reading books and articles, writing papers and carrying out research projects—must be one of the cornerstones on which good practice is founded.

4. One of the ways in which academic values can be engendered and fostered is through education—there must be more of it. One never hears doctors, psychologists or social workers talking about less education, they always want more: we have something to learn from them in that! We cannot hope to be accepted as equal partners in a teamwork approach unless we have something to offer—education will ensure that the community psychiatric nurse is fitted to take his place and hold his own in any company.

5. Team spirit! Everything leads up to it and everything flows from it. Community psychiatric nurses should aim to become and remain responsible members of the team, trained people conscious of their own abilities and potential, aware of the contribution they can make within the context of the team. Anything less will be bad for both patients and the nurses themselves, and not in society's interest.

THE WIDER CONTEXT

Under the Treaty of Rome, the U.K. in addition to its other links with the E.E.C., is tied in with the Community from the standpoint of health care practice as well. Comparability of standards of training are currently being looked at (cf. *Official Journal of the European Committees*, Volume **20**, No. L176: Council Decision 77/454/E.E.C.). We have a lot to offer the Community in the field of community psychiatric nursing and it seems certain that they will be interested in the experience and expertise developed over here already. The World Health Organisation has long advocated a 'community-based and -orientated (psychiatric) service', and sees the role of the nurse as 'vital', for she alone carries 24 hours, on-the-spot responsibility for patients'.(1)

Community psychiatric nursing services do exist in Europe: there is some interesting literature on the topic—cf. the U.S.S.R.(2,4), the Netherlands(3,4). (If readers are interested in a context wider even than that of the E.E.C. they may care to look at the following articles:

the U.S.A.(5,6) and Canada(7); plus of course the large number of articles already referred to in Chapter 7, all of which give some insights into developments in North America.)

There is little doubt that in the U.K. we have developed a long way in a relatively short time. We have amassed a variety of services and experience, developed training programmes and conducted major and minor research projects which must make us the envy of many. Whatever form the future takes on it certainly looks a bright one for community psychiatric nursing!

REFERENCES

1. W.H.O. Chronicle (1972) Trends in European psychiatric nursing care, *The Australian Nurses' Journal*, **2**, No. 1.
2. Carter, F. M. (1972) Community mental health services in the USSR, *Nursing Outlook*, **20**, No. 3.
3. Giel, R. (1974) A survey of psychiatric outpatient services in the province of Friesland (The Netherlands), *Tijdschrift Voor Sociale Geneeskunde*, **52**, No. 16.
4. Singer, P., Holloway, B., and Kolb, L. C. (1970) The psychiatrist-nurse team and home care in the Soviet Union and Amsterdam, *Journal of Psychiatric Nursing and Mental Health Services*, **8**.
5. Knight, I. (1976) The American experience, *Community Care*, August 18th.
6. Borus, J. F. (1976) Neighbourhood health centre as providers of primary mental health care, *The New England Journal of Medicine*, July 15th.
7. Cumming, J., Coates, D., and Bunton, P. (1976) Community care services in Vancouver: initial planning and implementation, *Canada's Mental Health*, **24**.

Index